Two Wolves
Collective
"The One You Feed"
Book I of V
The Book of Cub

Hunter W. Jones
Copyright © 2024 Hunter Jones
All rights reserved.
ISBN: 9798850433796

DEDICATION

"To my two wolves and higher self, GM, you have been walking next to me in my past, my present and long into the journey to come."

-Hunter W.J.

Also in the collection:

Book I: "The Book of Cub" - Laying the foundations of growth and self-discovery, focusing on the initial steps of personal development and overcoming basic challenges.

Book II: "The Omega's Journey" - Emphasizing the role of the individual within a larger community, focusing on building resilience, supporting others, and beginning to take on leadership roles.

Book III: "Delta: The Path of Growth" - Highlighting personal advancement and the development of intermediate skills, strategies, and insights necessary for leadership and advanced personal development.

Book IV: "Beta: The Leadership Forge" - Focused on honing leadership skills, influencing and guiding others, and preparing for the pinnacle of personal achievement and mastery.

Book V: "Alpha: The Mastery of Self" - Culminating the series, this book would explore achieving peak personal development, mastering self-discipline, leading with wisdom, and leaving a lasting impact on one's community and beyond.

CONTENTS

Pre challenge guide

CONTENTS

Wolf Cub: 30-day Challenge

Before we begin

I

Welcome, to the beginning of a journey unlike any other you've embarked on before. As you stand at the threshold of transformation, this book beckons you into a realm where ancient wisdom meets modern science, where the esoteric melds with the empirical, creating a tapestry of growth that is as profound as it is unique. You're about to dive into concepts and practices that may challenge your perceptions, stretch your boundaries, and invite you to explore the depths of your being. It's a path less trodden, sprinkled with the mystical, yet grounded in the tangible promise of self-renewal.

Embarking on this journey requires an open heart and an open mind. It demands trust in the system laid out before you—a system that, although unusual or entirely new to many, holds the keys to unlocking your fullest potential. If your body or mind resists, if skepticism whispers in your ear, I urge you to stick to the path. Give us just 30 days. Thirty days to gently guide you through a transformation that touches not just on health but on the very essence of what it means to live fully. I guarantee results that will not only surprise but also delight you.

This is not just a health book. It's a gateway to overcoming the hurdles of heartbreak, addiction, and procrastination. It's an all-encompassing blueprint for crafting the 'New You'—a version of yourself unburdened by the chains of past habits and freed to embrace the boundless possibilities of the present. This journey employs both modern and ancient techniques, embracing a holistic approach that may carry the fragrance of the esoteric, perhaps even hinting at the hippy, but rest assured, it packs a bite.

The beauty of this program lies in its simplicity. You need no equipment, no expensive subscriptions, just you, yourself, and the wolves that walk beside you (all will be explained). Whether you find yourself amidst the bustling city or the quiet countryside, this journey is tailor-made for you.

As you prepare to take this leap, know that you're not alone. A vibrant, supportive community awaits you, ready to share in your triumphs and offer comfort during challenges. I encourage you to join our Facebook and Instagram communities, where wisdom, encouragement, and stories of transformation are shared freely. Connect with us on Facebook at **facebook.com/2wolvescollective**. and follow us on Instagram at **@two.wolves.collective** to become part of a collective journey towards enlightenment and empowerment.

For those seeking a more personal connection or with specific inquiries, my inbox is always open. Reach out to me at **two.wolves.digital@gmail.com** with any questions, thoughts, or reflections. Your journey is deeply personal, but it is also part of a larger tapestry of collective healing and growth.

As you stand looking up at the mountain of change, ready to take that first step into the pages ahead, allow yourself to feel motivated, excited, and open to the transformation that awaits. This book is your guide, your mentor, and your map to a place where recovery, growth, and new beginnings are not just possible—they're guaranteed. Embrace this moment with joy and anticipation. The path to a new you, utilizing both the wisdom of ages and the insights of modern science, begins now. Let's walk this path together, with the wolves by our side, ready to emerge on the other side not just changed, but reborn.

Welcome to your journey. Welcome to the new you.
-Hunter W. Jones

The Legend of the Two Wolves

II

Long ago, in a remote forest, there lived a wise old Cherokee chief. He was known throughout the land for his wisdom and his ability to understand the ways of the world. One day, a young boy came to the old chief and asked, "What is your secret to living a happy and fulfilled life?" The old chief paused for a moment, then replied, "My dear child, there is a battle that rages within each of us, a battle between two wolves. One wolf is filled with anger, envy, sorrow, regret, greed, arrogance, self-pity, guilt, resentment, and ego. The other wolf is filled with love, joy, peace, kindness, compassion, generosity, empathy, faith, gratitude, and hope."

The young boy was confused and asked, "Which wolf will win the battle?" The old chief looked deep into the boy's eyes and said, "The one you feed." The boy was amazed by the wisdom of the old chief and he asked him how he could feed the good wolf and starve the bad one. The old chief explained that feeding the good wolf meant practicing acts of kindness, showing compassion to others, being grateful for the good things in life, and nurturing a positive attitude. He also explained that starving the bad wolf meant avoiding negative influences, such as gossip, anger, and jealousy, and letting go of the negative emotions that were holding the boy back. As the boy left, the old chief looked after him with a smile and a twinkle in his eye.

He knew that the boy had a long and difficult journey ahead of him, but he also knew that if the boy listened to his heart and followed the wisdom of the two wolves, he would find the happiness and fulfillment he sought.

And so the boy set out on his journey, filled with hope and determination, with the two wolves by his side. Together they faced the challenges of the forest, the obstacles that lay ahead, and the battles that raged within him.

But through it all, he kept his focus on the light wolf, feeding it with love and kindness, and letting go of the negative emotions that threatened to pull him down. In the end, the boy emerged victorious, having tamed the dark wolf and nurtured the light one. He knew that the battle would continue for the rest of his life, but he also knew that as long as he kept the two wolves in balance, he would always find the happiness and fulfillment he sought.

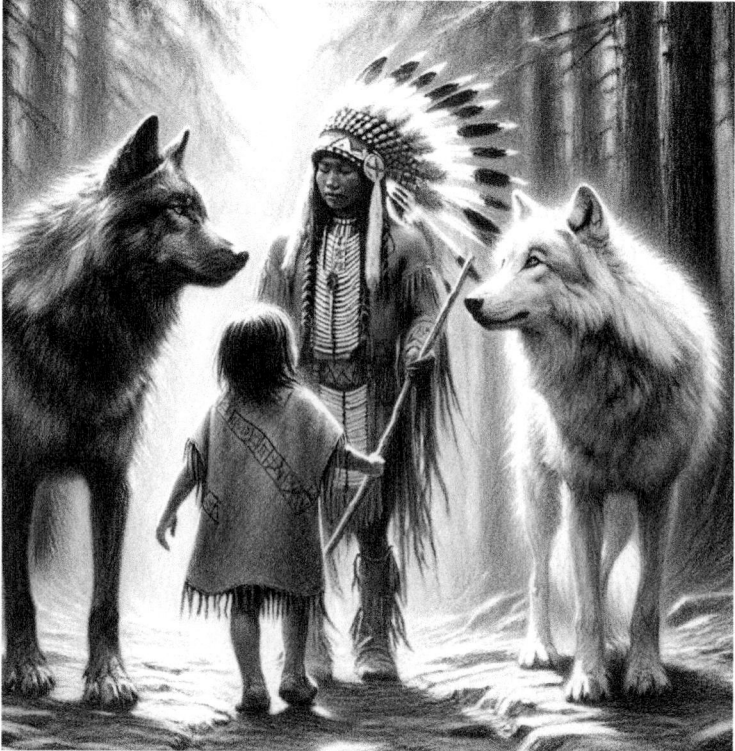

Introduction

III

Welcome to the Two Wolves Collective!

Embarking on this journey, you've taken a courageous step toward nurturing a healthier, more vibrant, and self-aware version of yourself. We are delighted to welcome you into our community, a place where each member embarks on a remarkable adventure of self-discovery and growth. The next 30 days promise to be an enriching period of challenge, enlightenment, and transformation.

This path is paved with opportunities for deep personal growth and the unveiling of your inner strengths. As we journey together, you'll find yourself amazed by your own evolution, equipped with the knowledge and habits to sustain your rejuvenated lifestyle.

Before we set off on this shared adventure, we encourage you to dive into the pre-program guide. This initial step is crucial as it lays the foundation for the transformative experiences to come. Take your time to absorb the insights, reflect on your intentions, and familiarize yourself with the practices that will soon become part of your daily life.

As you prepare to begin, remember that this journey is as much about the destination as it is about the journey itself. You are embarking on a path of self-discovery, armed with the power to reshape not only your physical well-being but also your mental and emotional landscapes.

"Please read the pre-30 day guide first, and when you are ready, we shall begin the journey. There's lots to cover, so shall we begin?"

Let this be a call to action, an invitation to step boldly into a space of transformation and empowerment. With every step, you will be feeding the wolf of courage, nurturing the positive, and learning to navigate the complexities of your inner world with grace and resilience.

"As we feed the wolf of courage, we silence the wolf of fear. Let us choose to nurture the positive and overcome the negative, for in the end, it is the wolf we feed that will win the fight." - **Hunter W.**

Are you ready to unfold the best version of yourself, to explore the depths of your potential, and to emerge from this journey transformed? Welcome to the beginning of your new chapter. Let's embark on this journey together, ready to embrace the challenges, celebrate the victories, and transform with every step we take.

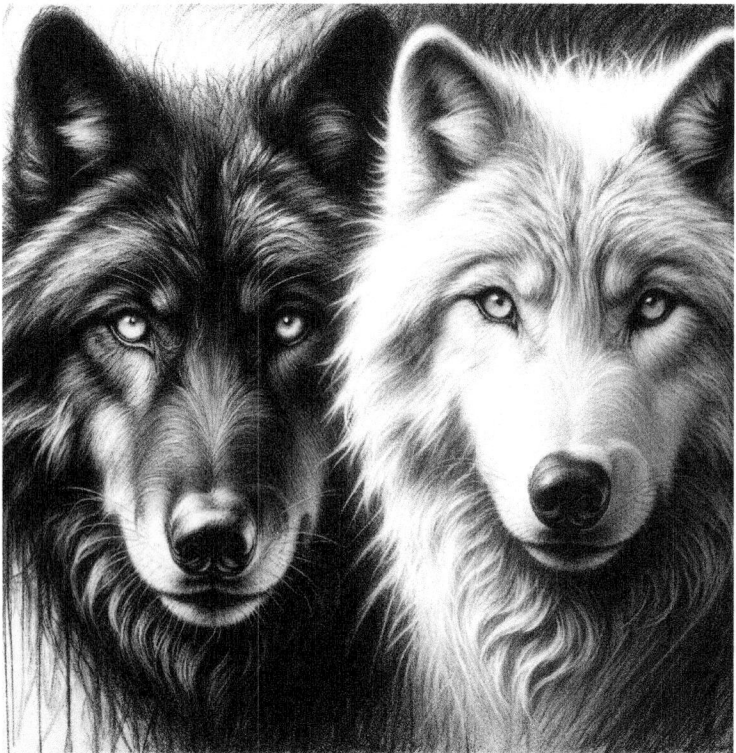

About the author

The genesis of the Two Wolves Collective is rooted deeply in the personal odyssey of Hunter, a man who once stood at the precipice of despair, his life unraveled by the challenges he faced. Hunter's journey through the darkest valleys of life, marked by battles with alcohol addiction, the loss of his company, and the dissolution of his marriage, is a testament to the human spirit's resilience and the transformative power of self-discovery.

At his lowest point, feeling disconnected from his true essence and ensnared by a web of negativity, Hunter stumbled upon the ancient wisdom of the two wolves—a philosophy that illuminates the duality within us all. One wolf embodies the shadows of fear, doubt, and negativity, while its counterpart radiates the light of positivity, hope, and courage. The philosophy holds that the wolf which thrives is the one we choose to nurture and feed.

This profound realization sparked a revolution within Hunter, guiding him to understand that the path to wellness is not just through the body but through the harmonious nurturing of the mind and spirit as well. Armed with this knowledge, Hunter embarked on creating a program that seamlessly integrates fitness, nutrition, and mindfulness, aiming to empower individuals to foster their inner light and silence the shadows.

With over 40 years of experience in entrepreneurship, coupled with internationally recognized certifications in personal training, nutrition, and wellness, Hunter brought invaluable insights and expertise to the formation of the Two Wolves Collective.

This journey, though fraught with obstacles, has been a beacon of transformation, not just for Hunter but for all who have been touched by the two wolves' philosophy.

Through the Two Wolves Collective, Hunter shares this powerful message of resilience and self-reinvention, inviting others to embark on their transformative journeys. It's an invitation to explore the depths of one's potential, to face life's adversities with courage, and to emerge not just victorious but transformed. Join us in embracing the ancient wisdom of the two wolves, and let it guide you towards a life of health, happiness, and fulfillment.

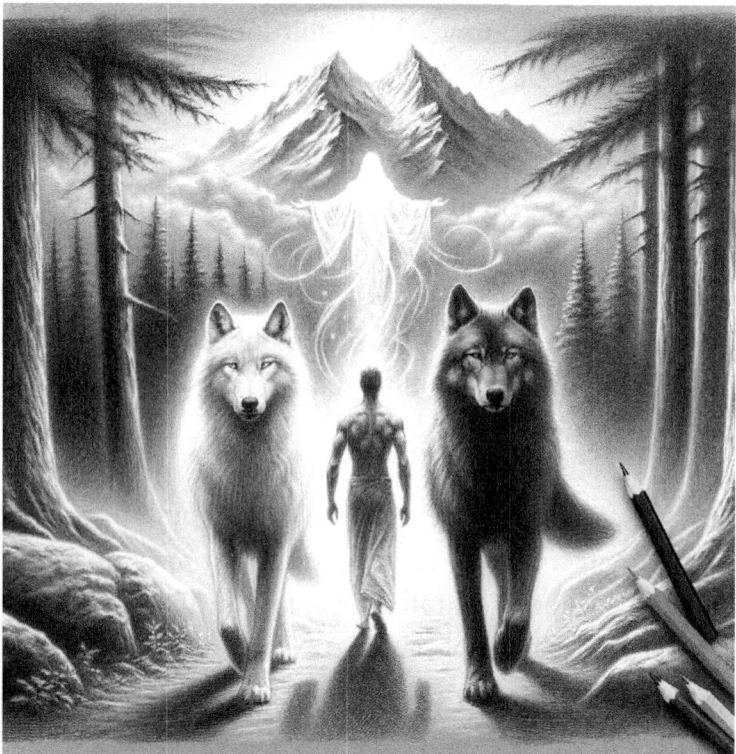

What is the Two Wolves Program?

V

The Two Wolves Collective harmonizes the prowess of modern technology with the profound depths of ancient spiritual beliefs and knowledge. This unique convergence crafts a transformative journey that guides individuals beyond the confines of their limitations, integrating the wisdom of the past with the innovations of the present to foster a holistic path to wellness and self-discovery.

Wolf Cubs: The Foundation (Book I of V)
The adventure commences with the Wolf Cubs stage, where the journey of transformation begins. This initial phase lays the foundational stones of physical health, nutritional understanding, and mental fortitude. Wolf Cubs are encouraged to cultivate positive habits, immerse themselves in the basics of physical fitness, and adopt a mindset ripe for growth and learning.

Omega Wolves: Building Resilience (Book II of V)
As participants evolve, they transition into the Omega Wolves phase, marking a critical period of strengthening and resilience-building. This stage emphasizes the development of endurance, both physical and mental, preparing participants for the intricate dynamics of the pack. Omega Wolves learn the importance of their role within the collective, focusing on the endurance and resilience necessary for the journey ahead.

Delta Wolves: Emerging Leadership (Book III of V)
Ascending to the Delta Wolves signifies the onset of leadership and mentorship.

Participants in this phase refine their leadership abilities, guiding and nurturing the growth of Wolf Cubs and Omega Wolves. This stage is about honing one's skills in physical and mental health and stepping into a role that requires guidance, wisdom, and the ability to inspire others.

Beta Wolves: The Pinnacle of Leadership (Book IV of V)
The Beta Wolves stand as the vanguard of the pack, assuming responsibility in guiding the collective in the Alpha's absence. This crucial phase sharpens strategic thinking, decision-making, and leadership skills. Beta Wolves refine their abilities to lead with integrity, inspire their peers, and embody the virtues of resilience and strength at the forefront of the pack.

Alpha Wolves: Mastery and Inspiration (Book V of V)
Reaching the Alpha Wolf stage symbolizes the zenith of one's journey within the Two Wolves Collective. Achieving this status is a testament to mastering physical fitness, mental agility, and leadership prowess. Alpha Wolves are the embodiment of the program's ultimate goals - to lead, inspire, and impact the lives of others positively. This phase celebrates the achievement of the highest level of self-realization, leadership, and the capacity to inspire change within the pack and beyond.

The Two Wolves Collective, with its blend of ancient wisdom and modern technology, offers a structured path through these stages, each designed to challenge, inspire, and elevate participants to new heights of personal achievement. This journey is not just about physical or mental transformation but about evolving into the best version of oneself through discipline, perseverance, and the support of a community that shares a common goal.

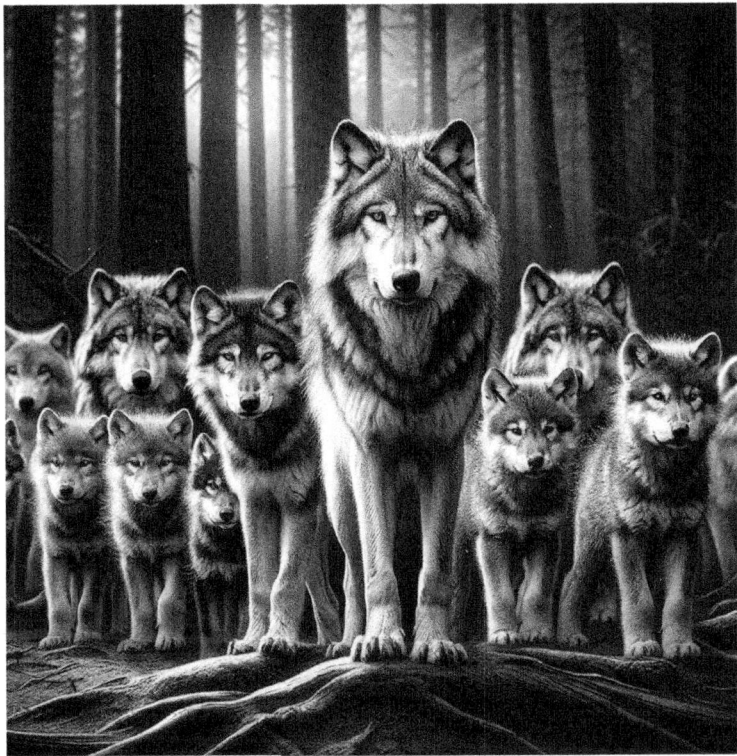

What is the Wolf Cub Program?

Embarking on the Two Wolves Collective, the first 30 days are encapsulated in "The Book of Cub," a comprehensive and transformative exploration aimed at sculpting the finest version of yourself. This phase of the journey seamlessly weaves together the essential strands of physical fitness, mental clarity, and nutritional enlightenment into a unified approach towards holistic wellness.

"The Book of Cub" is founded on the principle that meaningful transformation unfolds through a gradual, methodical process. Throughout this initial 30-day voyage, you'll engage with a carefully structured sequence of daily exercises and rituals crafted to establish a solid groundwork for your health and wellness odyssey.

Physical fitness is the cornerstone of this stage. With a balanced mix of steady-state cardio and calisthenics, the program is designed to bolster your strength, enhance your endurance, aid in fat reduction, and promote effective weight management. These exercises are intentionally challenging yet attainable, pushing you to expand your limits while ensuring an enjoyable and fulfilling experience.

Yet, **"The Book of Cub"** transcends physical boundaries, placing a significant emphasis on mental well-being. Through practices such as meditation and journaling, it cultivates a resilient and optimistic mindset, underscoring the inseparable link between mental health and physical vigor.

Nutrition is another fundamental aspect of this journey. Advocating for a diet rich in whole, nutrient-dense foods and steering clear of processed goods, high sugars, and refined carbohydrates, the program lays the nutritional foundation essential for sustaining health and wellness. This dietary approach is aimed at fueling your body with what it needs to thrive, supporting your transformation goals from the inside out.

"The Book of Cub" equips you with the knowledge, support, and tools necessary for a profound life transformation. It invites you to embrace this journey towards a healthier, more fulfilled you, grounded in the conviction that everyone has the potential to unlock their best selves. Let's go wolf cub, let's join your pack!

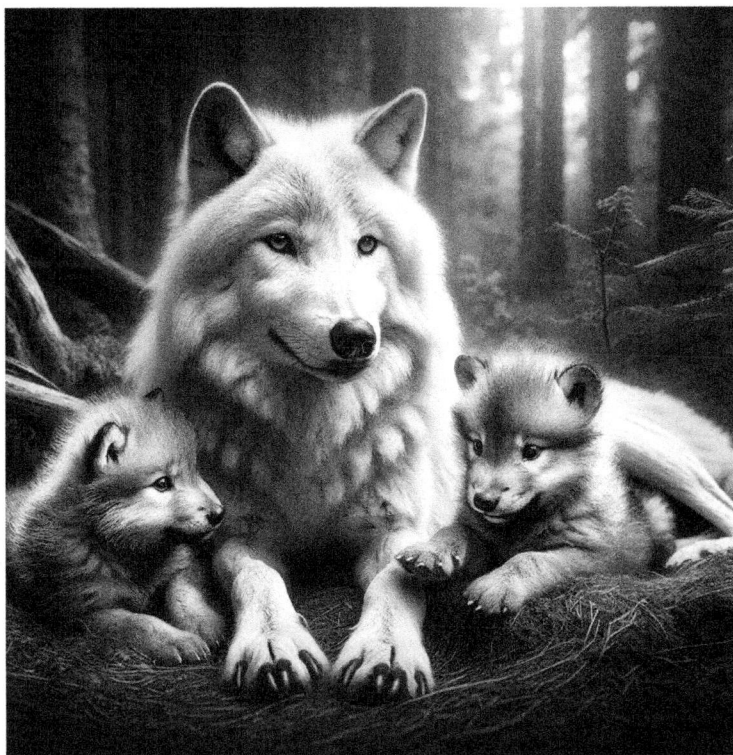

Phases of your journey

The Two Wolves philosophy intertwines the wisdom of ancient teachings with the insights of modern science, illustrating our capacity to guide our thoughts and actions. This philosophy forms the backbone of a 30-day program designed to nurture your inner strength, achieve equilibrium, and make enlightened choices by journeying through four distinct phases.

Phase 1: Foundations

In the initial week, known as the Foundations phase, you commence a journey of self-discovery and growth. This period is dedicated to establishing a solid base, integrating both new challenges and practices. You'll engage with exercises aimed at enhancing your physical strength, mental fortitude, and resilience, setting a precedent for the transformative experience ahead.

Phase 2: Transformations

The second week focuses on the inner battle with the dark wolf - the embodiment of self-sabotage and negative internal dialogue. Through a combination of physical exercises designed to push your boundaries and mindful practices like journaling and meditation, you'll confront and transform limiting beliefs. This phase harnesses the symbolic energy of the waxing moon, representing growth, to facilitate a shift from negative to positive states.

Phase 3: Empowerment

Empowerment week propels you into a state of heightened self-awareness and resilience. You'll explore themes such as conquering fear and anxiety, silencing your inner critic, cultivating self-compassion, enhancing adaptability, embracing mindful eating, managing stress, and fostering a supportive network.

This comprehensive approach, rooted in both ancient practices and contemporary psychological techniques, aims to arm you with the tools necessary for enduring empowerment.

Phase 4: Mastery
The final week, Mastery, is about consolidating your gains and pushing further into the realms of fitness and wellness. Focusing on endurance, stamina, and technique refinement, this phase also highlights the importance of rest, recovery, and the role of play in maintaining a balanced and healthy lifestyle. Here, the culmination of your efforts becomes evident, showcasing tangible results from the disciplined pursuit of personal excellence.

Through each phase, the Two Wolves program merges time-honored practices with the latest scientific research, offering a holistic path to personal transformation. This journey not only promises to reshape your physical and mental landscapes but also equips you with the knowledge and habits for a lifetime of wellness and self-realization.

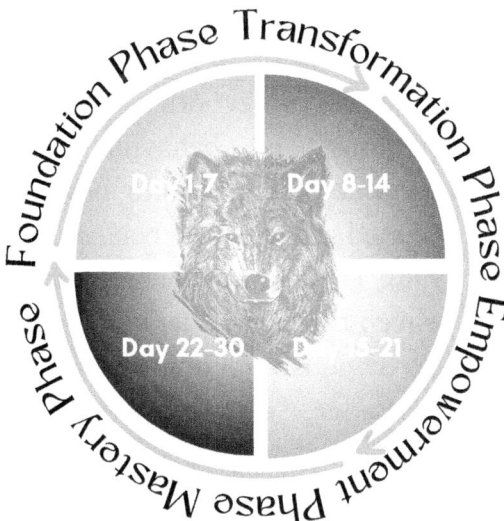

The Dark Wolf: Your Mind.

VIII

The foundational premise of the Two Wolves program is a deep exploration into the balance between two integral aspects of our psyche: the dark wolf, which symbolizes our negative emotions and inclinations, and the light wolf, represents our positive emotions and tendencies. This dichotomy within us is a fundamental aspect of our mental and emotional landscape, influencing our thoughts, actions, and overall state of well-being. The concept finds resonance in Carl Jung's work on the duality of human nature, where he posits that acknowledging our shadow is essential for achieving psychological integration ("Psychological Aspects of the Persona," 1938).

When we encounter internal debates—whether it's procrastinating on starting a healthier lifestyle or wrestling with feelings of self-worth—these are moments where the dark wolf asserts its presence. Such internal dialogues echo Freud's discussion of the id, the part of our psyche that drives our most primal impulses ("The Ego and the Id," 1923).

The dark wolf's persuasive power often leads us to reinforce negative thought patterns and behaviors, a process well-documented by neuroscience research into how our brains form and solidify patterns based on repeated behaviors (LeDoux, "The Emotional Brain," 1996). This reinforcement of negative patterns is a cycle that can be broken through understanding the principles of neuroplasticity, which demonstrate our brain's adaptability and capacity for change (Doidge, "The Brain That Changes Itself," 2007).

In countering the influence of the dark wolf, we draw upon the principles of psycho-cybernetics, a concept introduced by Maxwell Maltz. This theory posits that our self-image profoundly influences our behavior and that by altering our perception of ourselves, we can initiate significant changes in our lives ("Psycho-Cybernetics," 1960). The Two Wolves program incorporates this idea, emphasizing the development of a positive self-image as a means to empower individuals to make healthier choices and foster a more fulfilling life.

Furthermore, the work of Dr. Joe Dispenza offers insight into how understanding and modifying our thoughts and behaviors can lead to profound personal transformation. Dispenza's research into neuroplasticity and the quantum model of reality underscores the power of thought in shaping our lives and health ("Breaking the Habit of Being Yourself," 2012). By applying these principles, the Two Wolves program guides participants through the process of reshaping their self-image and, by extension, their reality.

The journey through the Two Wolves program is thus a comprehensive path that not only aims to tame the dark wolf but also to nourish the light wolf, advocating for a balanced coexistence of both. This approach is informed by both ancient wisdom and modern scientific insights, including the golden mean of Aristotelian ethics, which advocates for moderation and balance in all things (Aristotle, "Nicomachean Ethics," 4th Century BCE).

As participants embark on this transformative journey, they will engage with practices such as journaling, meditation, mindfulness, and physical challenges, all designed to build mental resilience and foster a positive self-image. Understanding your dark wolf, and not ignoring it is an integral part of this program. We do not run away from the dark, we sit in it until it becomes something that does not control us, but we control it!

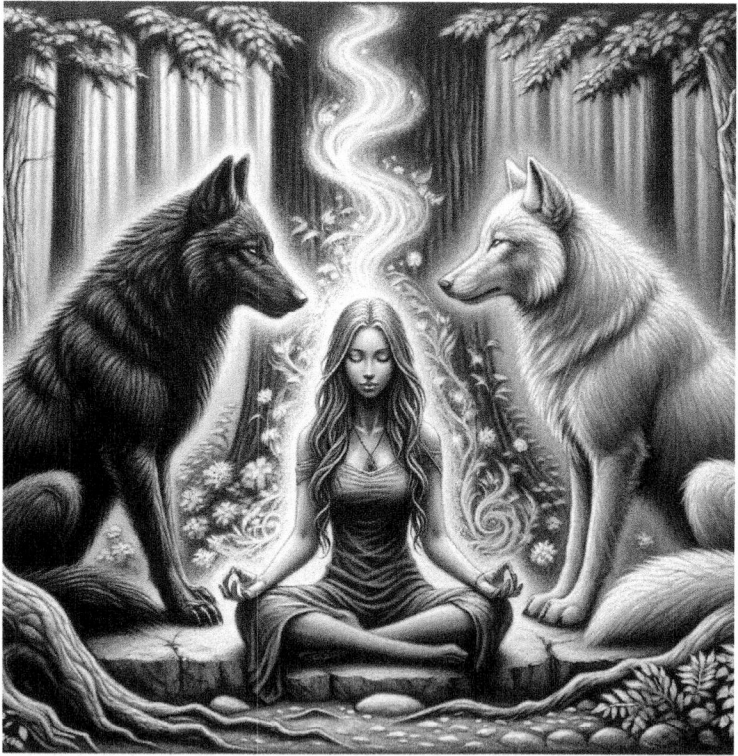

Our Mantra

IX

"move, breath, feed, believe, awoo"

Mantras serve as a potent tool in our psychological and emotional arsenal, acting as anchors or compasses that can guide us through the tumultuous seas of our minds. These concise, focused statements are more than mere words; they are imbued with the power to transform thoughts, influence behaviors, and recalibrate our emotional state. Research in cognitive behavioral therapy suggests that the repetitive use of positive affirmations can significantly impact our self-esteem, anxiety levels, and overall sense of well-being, essentially reprogramming the way we interact with our inner selves (Wood, Perunovic, & Lee, 2009).

Move The mantra "Move" is a call to action, a reminder of the vitality of physical activity for our mental and physical health. It's an acknowledgment that motion catalyzes emotion, where engaging in exercise can lead to a reduction in stress and an improvement in mood, as demonstrated in studies by Babyak et al. (2000). Saying or thinking "Move" propels us towards action, reinforcing the connection between an active body and a resilient mind.

Breathe "Breathe" centers us in the present moment, emphasizing the importance of mindful breathing in managing stress and anxiety. The act of focusing on our breath has been shown to lower stress levels and improve cognitive clarity (Ma et al., 2017). This mantra encourages us to pause, take a deep breath, and anchor ourselves in the now, facilitating a sense of calm and focus amidst life's chaos.

Feed "Feed" speaks to the necessity of nourishing our bodies with the right foods, recognizing the profound impact nutrition has on our overall well-being. Gómez-Pinilla (2008) highlights how nutrient-rich foods support brain function and energy levels. By reminding ourselves to "Feed," we commit to making choices that fuel our bodies optimally, ensuring we have the energy and health to pursue our goals.

Believe The mantra "Believe" taps into the transformative power of self-belief and positive thinking. This statement aligns with the principles of positive psychology, where a positive mindset is crucial for overcoming obstacles and achieving success (Seligman & Csikszentmihalyi, 2000). "Believe" serves as a self-affirmation, bolstering our confidence and reminding us of our capacity to manifest our aspirations.

Awoo Lastly, "Awoo" is our unique battle cry, a vocal expression that instantly sharpens our focus and reignites our purpose. This auditory cue, much like a wolf's howl, unites us in our collective and individual quests, symbolizing strength, direction, and camaraderie. The act of vocalizing "Awoo" can psychologically trigger a state of readiness and determination, preparing us to face our challenges head-on.

Each of these mantras plays a crucial role in the Two Wolves program, serving as daily reminders of our goals, values, and the strength we possess to achieve them. By integrating these mantras into our routine, either through thought or spoken word, we leverage their power to sculpt a path towards a balanced, fulfilled life.

Natural rhythm and balance

X

Our physiological and psychological well-being is intricately tied to the natural rhythms dictated by the sun's cycle. This circadian rhythm influences everything from our energy levels and mood to our cognitive capabilities. By aligning our daily activities with this inherent cycle, we unlock a powerful strategy to enhance our productivity and fulfill our aspirations with greater ease.

Dr. Andrew Huberman, a renowned neuroscientist at Stanford University, has shed light on the profound impact of light exposure on our brain's functioning. His pioneering research illustrates that morning exposure to sunlight can significantly bolster our circadian regulation, uplifting our mood, boosting energy, and sharpening our mental faculties. Conversely, evening exposure to blue light, especially from screens, can disrupt our sleep patterns and have adverse effects on our overall health.

To harness the full potential of our body's natural rhythm, adopting a daily routine synchronized with the sun's phases is key. Greeting the day with exposure to natural light, whether by stepping outdoors or utilizing a light therapy device, can invigorate us and prime us for a day filled with high-energy tasks and focused endeavors.

As the day unfolds, it's natural to experience a decline in energy and concentration. This period invites a transition to tasks of moderate intensity, providing an opportune moment for lighter activities, breaks, and physical movement to rejuvenate our minds and bodies.

The approach of evening signals a time to gradually unwind and prepare for restorative sleep. Minimizing blue light exposure from electronics, dimming household lights, and indulging in calming activities like reading or meditation can significantly enhance our sleep quality, making it easier to drift off and enjoy deeper rest.

Embracing the sun's rhythm requires a delicate balance between activity and relaxation, light and darkness. Incorporating both vigorous pursuits and periods of relaxation is essential for maintaining our overall performance and well-being. By understanding and adapting to our natural rhythms, we pave the way toward achieving a harmonious balance and realizing our utmost potential.

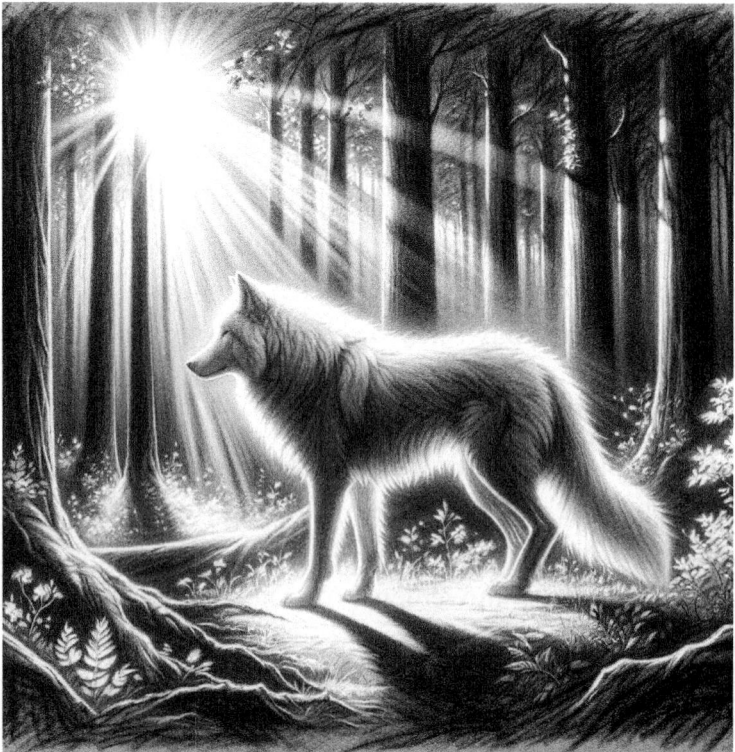

Your 10 Dailies & Trackers

As we stand at the threshold of the Book of Cub challenge, it's crucial to understand the foundation upon which this transformative journey is built. The 10 daily tasks outlined for you are not arbitrary; they are the pillars designed to support and guide your evolution in mind, body, and spirit. These tasks are rooted in principles of consistency, simplicity, and accountability—key elements that underpin the path to achieving the best version of yourself.

Consistency is the heartbeat of transformation. By engaging in these daily tasks, you establish a rhythm that nurtures gradual and sustainable change. It is through the repetition of positive behaviors that we can rewrite old patterns and cement new, healthier habits into our lives. Like the steady flow of water that shapes the hardest stone, consistency in your daily practices carves the path to profound personal growth.

Simplicity ensures that the journey is accessible and manageable. Each task has been distilled to its essence, focusing on fundamental actions that yield significant impacts. This approach demystifies the process of self-improvement, making it achievable for anyone willing to commit. Simplicity in our daily tasks removes the barrier of complexity, allowing us to concentrate on the essence of transformation with clarity and purpose.

Accountability stands as the framework that supports your commitment to this challenge. Sharing your journey with "The Pack", tracking your progress, and engaging with daily educational assignments not only foster a sense of community but also reinforce your responsibility to yourself and others.

Accountability magnifies the impact of your efforts, turning individual pursuits into a shared journey of empowerment and collective achievement.

Now, as we introduce the daily tasks, remember that these practices are carefully curated to catalyze your transformation:

1. **Movement**: Achieve 10,000 steps daily, fostering physical vitality.
2. **Mindfulness** Meditation: Dedicate 15 minutes to meditation, utilizing Hunter W.'s YouTube channel for guidance.
3. **The Wolf Workout:** Participate in the structured Wolf Workout, enhancing strength and endurance.
4. **Hydration**: Drink 4 liters of water a day, ensuring optimal hydration.
5. **When to feed:** Follow an 8-hour eating window, integrating fasting for health benefits.
6. **Packwork**: Complete educational tasks to expand your wellness knowledge.
7. **Supplementation**: [Optional] Use supplements to support nutritional well-being.
8. **Sleep**: Prioritize 7-9 hours of sleep for recovery and rejuvenation.
9. **Progress Tracking**: Document your journey with daily photos, observing your transformation.
10. **What to feed on**: Eliminate alcohol and processed foods, embracing a clean diet.

As you embark on this journey, embrace these tasks with an understanding of their purpose and the principles they embody. Consistency, simplicity, and accountability are your allies on this path, guiding you towards a holistic transformation. Together, let's step forward into this adventure, ready to unfold the greatest version of yourself.

Daily 1: Movement

Walking, a fundamental human activity, resonates deeply with our evolutionary history. It's a practice that has sustained us for millennia, not just as a mode of transportation but as a vital component of our health and well-being. The goal of walking 10,000 steps a day, while seemingly modern, taps into this ancestral practice, offering numerous benefits that extend far beyond simple locomotion.

"Walking is the best possible exercise. Habituate yourself to walk very far," advised Thomas Jefferson, highlighting the timeless value of this simple activity. In today's era, where sedentary lifestyles predominate, the act of walking becomes even more crucial. It serves as an antidote to the hours spent in stationary positions, actively combating the health detriments of a sedentary life. As a form of low-impact exercise, walking is universally accessible, requiring no special equipment or environment, making it an ideal activity for individuals across all fitness levels.

The mental health benefits of walking are equally compelling. Research has consistently shown that regular walking can significantly reduce symptoms of anxiety and depression, providing a natural and accessible mood booster. *"In every walk with nature, one receives far more than he seeks,"* John Muir famously stated, encapsulating the mental and emotional rejuvenation that comes from stepping into the outdoors. The act of walking allows for a momentary retreat from the digital world, offering a chance to reconnect with the environment and oneself, fostering a sense of tranquility and present-mindedness.

Within the Two Wolves program, walking is championed not only as a physical exercise but as a meditative and restorative practice. Encouraging participants to achieve 10,000 steps daily is more than a fitness goal; it's an invitation to embrace a lifestyle change that nurtures both body and mind. This commitment to daily walking can catalyze significant improvements in physical health, enhance mental well-being, and lay the foundation for a lifelong habit of movement and mindfulness.

By integrating walking into our daily routine, we embark on a path towards enhanced fitness, diminished stress, and a deeper connection with the natural world. It is a simple yet profoundly effective way to cultivate health, happiness, and well-being, embodying the essence of the Two Wolves program's holistic approach to personal transformation.

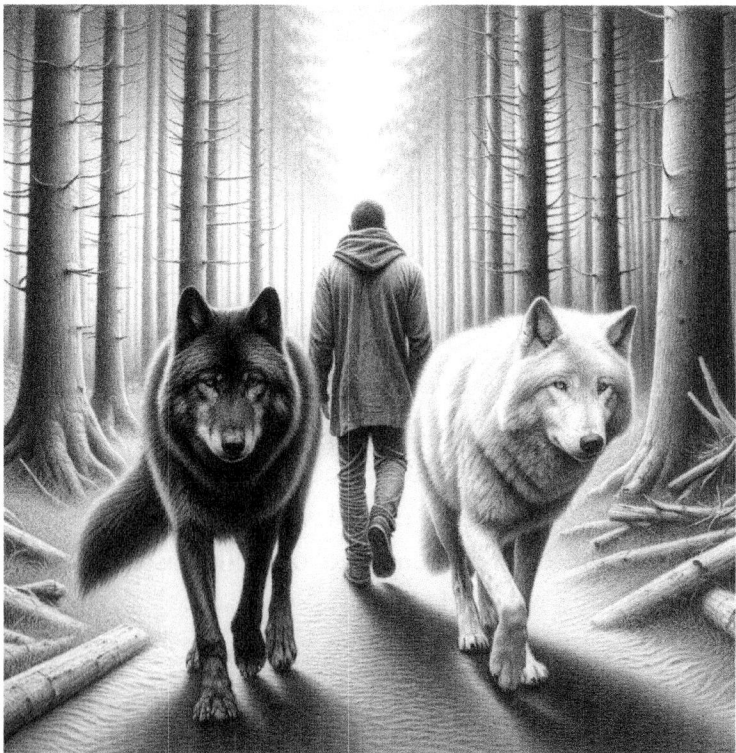

Daily 2: Mindfulness

The core of the Two Wolves program lies not just in the practice of meditation but in the profound journey of self-discovery it initiates. This journey invites us to confront and engage with the two wolves within us, representing the duality of our nature. It is a profound exploration of who we are at our very essence and the internal forces that shape our thoughts, behaviors, and ultimately, our lives. This meditation practice, diligently followed for 30 days, is not merely a routine but a voyage into the depths of our being, where true transformation begins.

At the heart of this transformative journey is the concept of neuroplasticity, championed by figures like Dr. Joe Dispenza. Neuroplasticity offers us the scientific foundation to understand how meditation can fundamentally alter our brain's structure and function, leading to lasting changes in our thoughts, emotions, and behaviors. *"You are not doomed by your genes and hardwired to be a certain way for the rest of your life,"* Dispenza writes, emphasizing our capacity for change ("You Are the Placebo"). By engaging in meditation, we leverage this incredible ability of our brains to rewire and evolve, guiding ourselves toward the best versions of who we can be.

Confronting the two wolves within us through meditation is an act of profound courage and introspection. It requires us to acknowledge the presence of our dark wolf, the embodiment of our fears, insecurities, and negative patterns, and to recognize the power of our light wolf, the source of our strengths, hopes, and positive aspirations. This process is akin to the ancient practice of self-examination, a philosophical undertaking noted by Socrates when he declared, *"The unexamined life is not worth living."*

The daily engagement with our meditations, accessible to all through the Two Wolves YouTube channel *(link on the links page at the back of the book)*, provides a structured pathway for this exploration. Each session is designed to deepen your understanding of the two wolves and their influence on your life. Through consistent practice, you gradually learn to communicate with these internal aspects, transforming your relationship with yourself and fostering a sense of harmony and balance.

This meditation journey is fundamentally about transformation—transforming not just our minds but our entire beings. As we learn to communicate with and understand our two wolves, we uncover insights about our deepest desires, fears, and potentials. This knowledge is power—the power to shape our lives in alignment with our true selves and to manifest the reality we aspire to.

Integrating this meditation practice into your daily life, alongside the other healthful habits promoted in the Two Wolves program, sets the stage for a comprehensive transformation. It supports not only the achievement of physical health and mental clarity but also the cultivation of a life lived with intention, purpose, and authenticity.

In embracing this journey, you are doing more than adopting a new routine; you are embarking on a path of profound self-discovery and growth. By confronting and engaging with your two wolves, you unlock the potential to transform into the best version of yourself, armed with a deeper understanding of who you are and the incredible capability you have to shape your destiny.

Mindfulness (additional)

Shadow Work: Embracing Our Whole Self

Shadow work, a concept introduced by Carl Jung, involves confronting the parts of ourselves that we've denied or suppressed —the "shadow." These aspects, though often perceived as negative, hold the key to our wholeness and authenticity. Meditation provides a safe space for this exploration, allowing us to observe and integrate these hidden parts with compassion and without judgment. As Jung famously said, "One does not become enlightened by imagining figures of light, but by making the darkness conscious." Through consistent practice, we learn to acknowledge and embrace our entire being, unlocking a deeper understanding of ourselves and fostering genuine self-acceptance.

Detachment Theory: The Freedom to Let Go

Detachment theory, often explored in Buddhist philosophy, teaches the liberating power of releasing our attachment to outcomes, people, and the myriad desires that tether us to suffering. Meditation cultivates a state of detached observation, where we learn to witness our thoughts and emotions without getting entangled. This practice of non-attachment doesn't mean disconnection or apathy but rather finding freedom in the present moment, unburdened by the past or future.

It's in this space of detachment that we find the strength to heal a broken heart, embracing our experiences without letting them define us.

The Art of Letting Go: Transformation through Release

The ability to let go is intrinsically linked to our capacity for change and growth. Letting go of old patterns, beliefs, and fears is essential in making room for new possibilities. Meditation serves as a powerful tool in this process, facilitating moments of quiet reflection where we can gently release what no longer serves us. As we cultivate this practice with consistency, we find that letting go becomes less about loss and more about opening ourselves to new horizons and opportunities.

Meditation: A Catalyst for Healing and Becoming

At its core, meditation is about presence, awareness, and the intentional redirection of our focus. For those navigating the pain of a broken heart or the desire to reinvent themselves, meditation offers a path to clarity and motivation. It helps us to dissolve the barriers of fear and doubt, illuminating the strength and resilience within. By committing to this practice daily, we embrace the principles of simplicity, consistency, and accountability, each step forward guided by the inner wisdom that emerges in stillness.

In summary, meditation is not merely a practice but a journey back to ourselves, through the valleys of shadow work, the peaks of detachment, and the rivers of letting go. It's a journey that demands courage, commitment, and the willingness to confront and embrace all facets of our being. By integrating meditation into our daily routine, we embark on a transformative path, one that heals, empowers, and reveals the limitless potential that lies within. All the guided meditations you need can be found on the dedicated Two Wolves Collective youtube channel:

Daily 3: The Wolf Workouts

Welcome to the transformative world of the Two Wolves program, where the 'Wolf Workouts' await to revolutionize your physical conditioning. Tailored for everyone, regardless of age, gender, or fitness level, these callisthenic exercises embody the principles of consistency, simplicity, and accountability, ensuring they can be seamlessly integrated into your daily life.

The essence of the Wolf Workouts lies in their straightforward yet impactful design. Here's a glimpse into the regimen:

1. **5x5 Body Squat:** A cornerstone for lower body strength, focusing on form to target key muscle groups.
2. **5x5 Push-Up:** A fundamental upper-body exercise that enhances strength across the chest, triceps, and shoulders.
3. **5x5 Leg Raise:** Targets the lower abdominals for core strengthening with precision and control.
4. **5x30s Elbow Plank**: Bolsters core stability by engaging multiple muscle groups in a sustained hold.
5. **5x5 Step Up:** Enhances lower body and cardiovascular health through repetitive motion.

To ensure your success and progression, each workout is designed to evolve weekly, gradually intensifying by adding repetitions and extending plank durations. This methodical increase not only promotes physical improvement but also keeps you engaged and motivated.

The key to unlocking the full potential of these workouts is rooted in consistency; dedicating yourself to perform these exercises daily lays the groundwork for significant transformation. Simplicity in the structure of the workouts ensures they are accessible and manageable, allowing you to focus on form and technique without the need for complex equipment or facilities.

Lastly, accountability plays a critical role; by tracking your progress and possibly sharing your journey with our community, you reinforce your commitment to your fitness goals.

In the forthcoming pages, I will dive deeper into the specifics of how to execute each exercise with optimal efficiency and safety. This detailed guidance is designed to equip you with the knowledge to perform each movement correctly, maximizing the benefits while minimizing the risk of injury.

Embrace these workouts with the spirit of a wolf — with determination, resilience, and the pursuit of excellence. Consistency, simplicity, and accountability are your allies on this journey towards physical empowerment. Let's embark on this path together, transforming not just the body, but the mind and spirit as well, as you grow stronger with every rep, every step, and every breath.

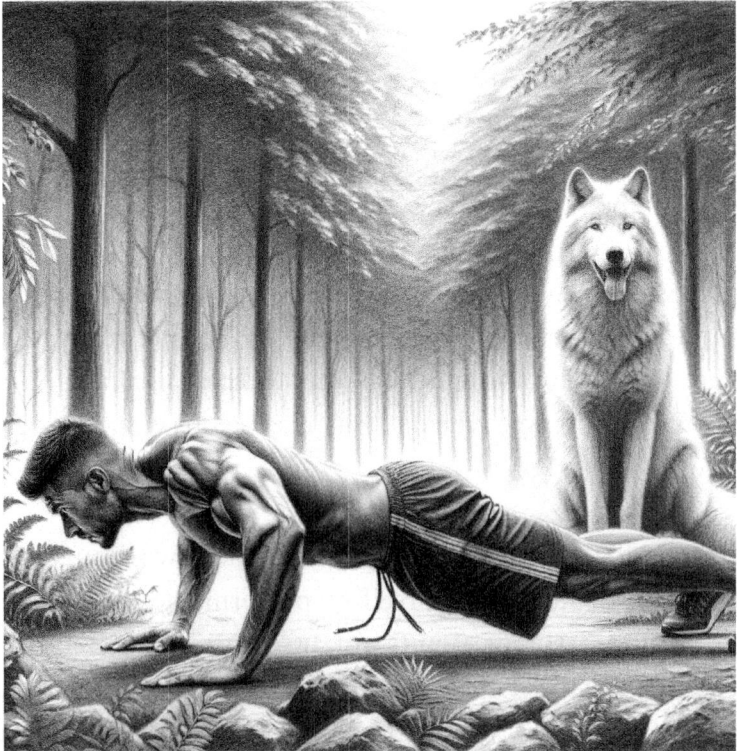

The Wolf Workouts: Body Squat

Squats are an essential exercise that works several key muscle groups, including your quadriceps, hamstrings, glutes, and core. To avoid injury and maximize benefits, it's crucial to squat with proper form. Here's a simplified guide to executing a correct squat:

1. **Position:** Stand with feet hip-width apart, toes angled slightly outwards.
2. **Core Engagement:** Tighten your core by drawing your belly button toward your spine.
3. **Descent:** Initiate the squat by pushing your hips back and bending at the knees, as if sitting down in an invisible chair.
4. **Depth:** Lower yourself until your thighs are at least parallel to the floor, maintaining knee alignment with your toes.
5. **Ascent:** Push through your heels to stand back up, keeping your core tight and back straight throughout the movement.

Additional Tips for a Flawless Squat:

- Ensure your knees stay aligned with your toes and resist the urge to let them collapse inward.
- Maintain an upright chest and a neutral spine from start to finish.
- Focus on pushing up from your heels to engage the correct muscles.
- Begin with bodyweight squats; as your technique improves, gradually introduce weights to increase challenge.

Adhering to these steps and tips will help you perform squats safely and effectively, tapping into the full potential of this comprehensive exercise.

1.

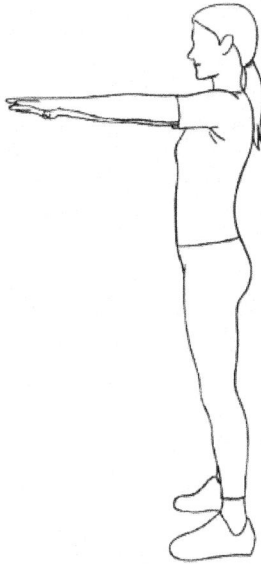

2.

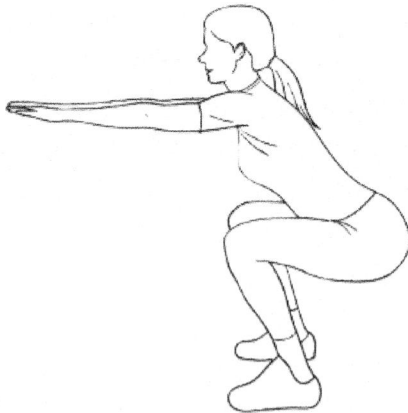

The Wolf Workouts: Push Up

Push-ups are an excellent compound exercise that targets the chest, arms, shoulders, and core, offering a full-body workout. To ensure you reap the maximum benefits while minimizing the risk of injury, follow these streamlined steps for a proper push-up:

1. **Starting Position**: Begin in a plank stance, hands shoulder-width apart directly under your shoulders, and feet hip-width apart. Your body should form a straight line from head to heels.
2. **Descent**: Gradually lower your body, aiming to get your chest close to the ground. Keep your elbows tucked in to engage the target muscles effectively. Ensure your body maintains a straight line, engaging your core to support your posture.
3. **Ascent**: Press down through your palms, extending your arms to lift yourself back to the starting plank position. Keep your body aligned and straight throughout this movement.
4. **Repetition**: Continue the exercise for your set number of repetitions, maintaining form and alignment with each push-up.

Effective Push-Up Tips:
- Ensure your elbows stay close to your sides to maximize engagement across your chest, triceps, and shoulders.
- Activate your core throughout the push-up to support your spine and enhance stability.
- Maintain a neutral neck by focusing your gaze slightly ahead on the floor, avoiding straining your neck by looking up or letting your head droop.
- Coordinate your breath with the movement: inhale on the descent and exhale on the ascent.

For beginners or those building strength, starting with modified push-ups on your knees is a sensible approach. As your strength and confidence grow, you can transition to full push-ups. Consistent practice with attention to form will lead to noticeable improvements in strength and endurance, making push-ups a cornerstone of your workout regimen.

1.

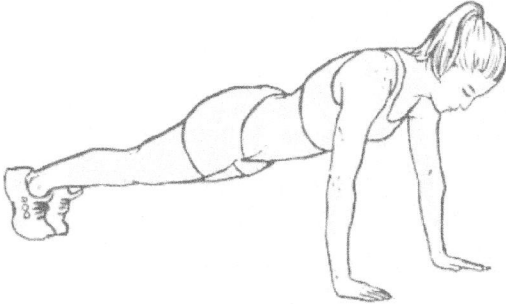

2.

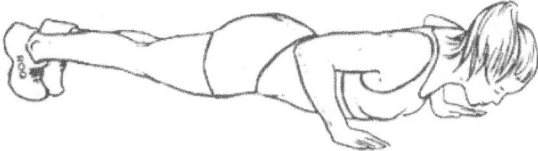

The Wolf Workouts:
Leg Raise

Leg raises are an effective exercise for fortifying your core, specifically targeting the lower abdominal muscles. Follow these detailed steps to ensure you're performing leg raises with precision and safety:

1. **Positioning**: Start by lying flat on your back on a comfortable exercise mat or the floor. Extend your legs fully in front of you, keeping your feet together.
2. **Support**: Slide your hands, palms down, under your glutes. This position helps provide stability to your lower back throughout the exercise.
3. **Core Engagement**: Take a deep breath in, simultaneously drawing your belly button towards your spine to activate your core muscles firmly.
4. **Lifting**: With your legs kept straight, gradually elevate them off the floor, aiming to form a 90-degree angle with your torso. The movement should be controlled and deliberate.
5. **Peak Hold**: Once your legs reach the vertical position, pause briefly to intensify the engagement of your lower abs.
6. **Descent**: Gently lower your legs back to the starting position, maintaining control and keeping your core engaged.
7. **Breathing**: Exhale as you lift your legs and inhale on the return. This breathing pattern aids in maintaining core engagement and stability.

Additional Leg Raise Tips:
- Strive to keep your legs as straight as possible throughout the exercise to maximize the efficacy of the movement.
- Ensure your lower back remains in contact with the mat, preventing any arching that could lead to strain.

- Avoid relying on momentum to lift your legs; the power should come from your core, specifically your lower abdominals.
- Should you experience any discomfort or pain in your lower back, cease the exercise and seek guidance from a fitness or medical professional.

By adhering to these instructions, leg raises can significantly enhance your core strength, offering benefits to your overall fitness level and physical health.

1.

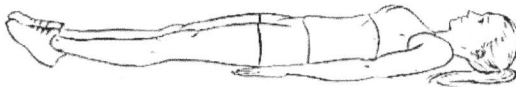

2.

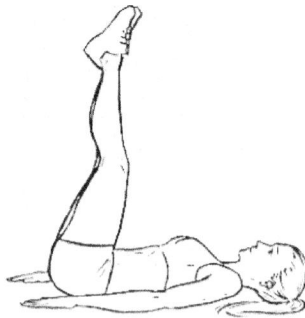

The Wolf Workouts: Elbow Plank

The elbow plank is an excellent core-strengthening exercise that targets your abdominals, back, and hips, enhancing stability and posture. To perform an elbow plank with precision, follow these streamlined steps:

1. **Initial Position**: Lie face down on an exercise mat or a comfortable surface, preparing for the movement.
2. **Elbow Alignment:** Place your elbows beneath your shoulders, ensuring they are aligned correctly. Rest your forearms on the ground, forming fists with your hands.
3. **Leg Extension:** Stretch your legs out behind you, keeping your feet together and toes tucked under, ready to engage your core.
4. **Lift and Tighten:** Activate your abdominal muscles and glutes, lifting your torso off the ground. Aim to create a straight line from your head to your heels, keeping your back flat and hips even.
5. **Duration:** Hold this position with controlled breathing for at least 30 seconds initially, challenging yourself to maintain form and stability.
6. **Release:** To conclude, carefully lower your body back to the mat, returning to your starting position.

Effective Elbow Plank Tips:
- Ensure your shoulders are positioned away from your ears to maintain a neutral neck alignment.
- Deeply engage your core by pulling your belly button toward your spine, fortifying the plank's effectiveness.
- Keep your body in a straight alignment, preventing your hips from dipping or arching.

- Focus on deep, even breaths to support core engagement and endurance throughout the hold.
- Gradually extend the duration of your plank as your core strength builds, ensuring continuous improvement.

Mastering the elbow plank with proper form is crucial for harnessing its full benefits and laying a foundation for more advanced core exercises. Prioritize technique and gradual progress to strengthen your core effectively and safely.

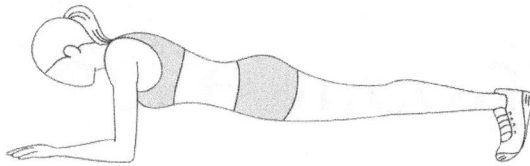

The Wolf Workouts: The Step Up

Step-ups are an effective lower body exercise that primarily engages the glutes, quads, and hamstrings. Here's how to execute step-ups with proper technique:

1. **Equipment Selection:** Choose a sturdy platform, such as a box or step, that reaches about knee height or slightly above.
2. **Starting Position:** Position yourself in front of the selected platform with your feet hip-width apart. Let your arms hang naturally by your sides.
3. **Initial Step:** Place your right foot entirely on the platform, ensuring the whole foot is securely positioned, including the heel.
4. **Ascent:** Drive through your right foot, engaging your glutes and thigh muscles to bring your left foot up, achieving a standing position atop the platform.
5. **Descent:** Carefully step back down with your left foot, followed by your right, returning to your original stance.
6. **Repetition:** Complete the set number of repetitions, then switch your leading foot to the left and repeat the sequence.

Effective Step-Up Tips:
- Maintain an upright posture with your chest lifted and core braced throughout the movement to ensure stability and alignment.
- Keep your stepping knee in direct alignment with your toes, avoiding any inward collapse which can strain the knee.
- Focus on utilizing your glute muscles to power the step-up motion and control your movement as you descend.

- Begin with a lower height to master the form. As your strength and confidence grow, you can gradually increase the platform's height for an added challenge.
- Should you feel any discomfort in your knees, halt the exercise immediately. Consider consulting a fitness professional to ensure you're performing the movement correctly or to adjust the exercise to better suit your needs.

Mastering step-ups with proper form is crucial for maximizing the exercise's benefits while minimizing the risk of injury. By following these guidelines, you'll effectively strengthen your lower body in a safe and progressive manner.

1. **2.**

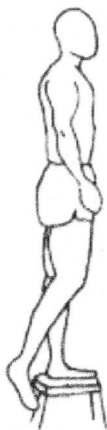 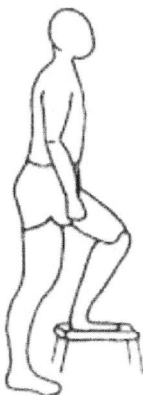

Daily 4: Hydration

Incorporating a daily intake of 4 liters (approximately 1 gallon) of water is a cornerstone of the Two Wolves program, underscoring water's vital role in maintaining optimal health. Water serves as the lifeblood of our physiological processes, facilitating nutrient and oxygen delivery to cells, regulating temperature, and purging toxins and waste from our body. The repercussions of inadequate hydration extend beyond mere thirst, manifesting as headaches, fatigue, and diminished physical and cognitive performance.

Committing to this hydration goal is integral to achieving your wellness objectives. Regular, ample water consumption not only ensures hydration but also aids in detoxifying your body and promoting efficient digestive function. Moreover, staying well-hydrated can temper appetite, assisting in nutritional discipline and weight management efforts.

Adopting practical strategies can simplify meeting your daily water intake target. Keeping a refillable water bottle at hand allows for convenient hydration throughout the day. Establishing reminders to drink water at regular intervals, beginning your day with a glass of water, and hydrating before meals can further embed this healthy habit into your routine. For an added twist, consider infusing your water with slices of fruits or herbs, enhancing its flavor and making hydration an enjoyable ritual.

Hydration is not merely a recommendation within the Two Wolves program—it's imperative for unlocking your full health and fitness potential. By prioritizing a gallon of water daily, you're not just quenching thirst but paving the way for physical well-being and advancing towards your fitness milestones.

Daily 5: Time to feed

Mastering nutrition is pivotal to the success of your 30-day challenge within the Two Wolves program, standing as a critical pillar in your journey towards transformation. Given the complexity of nutrition science, the program simplifies this area into actionable, straightforward principles, ensuring it's approachable yet profoundly effective.

Key Nutritional Guidelines for the Cub Program:
1. **Eliminate Cheat Meals:** For the next 30 days, steer clear of processed foods and sugary indulgences. These items often fall under the influence of the 'Dark Wolf' — the internal force driving poor dietary choices. Recognizing this can empower you to make healthier decisions.
2. **Abstain from Alcohol:** Alcohol can disrupt your sleep patterns and hydration, adversely affecting both physical and mental performance. Its elimination is essential for maintaining focus and discipline throughout the program.
3. **Adopt an 8-Hour Eating Window:** This intermittent fasting approach is a cornerstone of the program, encouraging discipline while offering significant health benefits. Condensing your eating to an 8-hour period promotes better insulin sensitivity, reduces inflammation, and enhances cellular repair, according to emerging nutritional science.
4. **Practice Logical Portion Control:** Aim for balanced meals with adequate protein (roughly the size of your fist), complemented by abundant non-starchy vegetables. This method helps in avoiding overeating while ensuring you're nourished with the essential nutrients.

Implementing These Practices:

By focusing your diet on whole foods, you provide your body with the necessary fuel for optimal function. Embrace a variety of proteins, healthy fats, and complex carbohydrates to keep your meals balanced and satisfying. Avoid the temptation of processed and fast foods, which can derail your progress.

Intermittent fasting, or eating within an 8-hour window, not only simplifies your dietary routine but also aligns with the body's natural rhythms, supporting weight management and overall health. This approach, coupled with mindful portion control, forms a solid foundation for lasting dietary habits.

Support and Inspiration:

To further support your journey through the Two Wolves program and ensure you have all the tools necessary for success, we've created the "Two Wolves Cookbook." This comprehensive guide is filled with recipes that align perfectly with the nutritional principles outlined in the program, from whole foods to balanced meals that fit within your 8-hour eating window. Each recipe is designed not only to nourish your body but also to satisfy your taste buds, making healthy eating both enjoyable and sustainable.

Whether you're seeking inspiration for quick breakfasts, nutritious lunches, wholesome dinners, or healthy snacks, the "Two Wolves Cookbook" has you covered. With options catering to various dietary preferences, you'll find meals that support your health goals while adding variety to your daily routine.

To purchase your copy of the "Two Wolves Cookbook" and embark on a culinary adventure that complements your fitness journey, visit the following link: [Link Page at the back of this book].

Understanding the Science:

Recent studies underscore the effectiveness of intermittent fasting and a whole-food diet in enhancing health outcomes. Improved insulin sensitivity, better body composition, and reduced inflammation are just a few of the benefits documented in the scientific literature (Varady et al., 2019; Willett et al., 2019).

As we delve deeper in the following chapters, you'll gain a comprehensive understanding of why these nutritional strategies are essential in the Two Wolves program. Nutrition isn't just about fueling the body; it's about nourishing the soul and embracing a lifestyle that brings out the best in you.

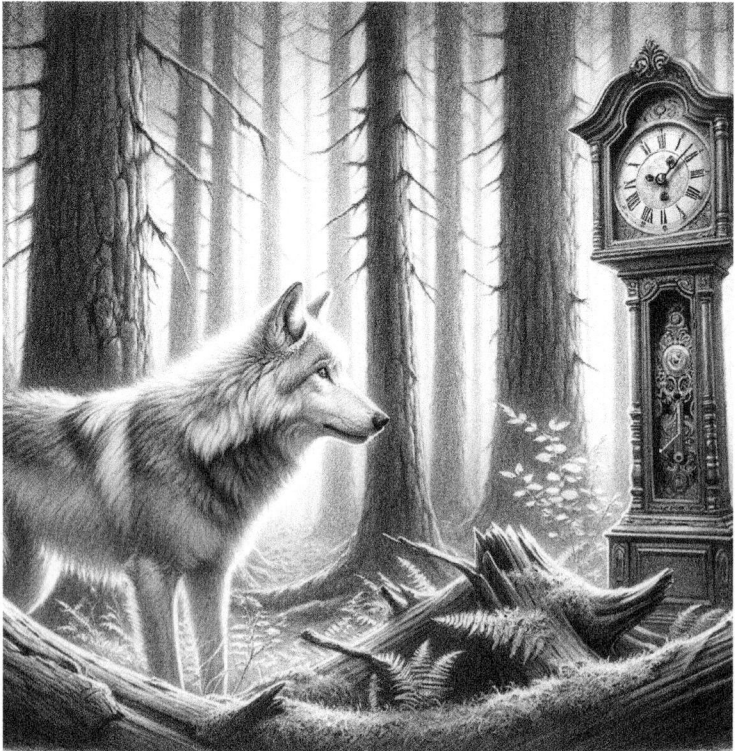

Daily 6: What to feed on

Embarking on the Two Wolves program is not just a commitment to physical fitness; it's an invitation to a holistic transformation that touches every aspect of your being. At the core of this journey is the ancient wisdom encapsulated in the tale of the Two Wolves, a narrative that teaches us about the dual nature within each of us— the 'good wolf' that thrives on joy, peace, and love, and the 'dark wolf' that feeds on fear, anger, and resentment. This chapter delves into how our daily choices, particularly in nutrition, directly influence which wolf we nurture and how mindfulness and the strength of our community can guide us toward our truest selves.

Feeding the Good Wolf Through Nutrition
Understanding nutrition as a fundamental element of this program requires recognizing the literal and metaphorical significance of 'the one you feed.' Every meal, every bite, and every dietary choice is an opportunity to either nourish the good wolf within us, promoting health, vitality, and wellness, or to inadvertently give strength to the dark wolf, leading us down a path of diminished health and disconnection from our true needs.

1. **Whole Foods Over Fast Food and Alcohol:** In choosing whole foods rich in nutrients over fast food laden with unhealthy fats, sugars, and excessive salt, we make a conscious decision to feed the good wolf. The adverse effects of fast food and alcohol consumption are well-documented, linked to chronic health issues, impaired mental function, and a disrupted emotional balance. Opting for nourishment that supports our body's needs is a step toward resilience, clarity, and a deeper connection with ourselves.

- **The Power of Intermittent Fasting:** Adopting an 8-hour eating window is not just about discipline; it's about aligning with our body's natural rhythms, enhancing metabolic health, and fostering a mindful relationship with food. This practice, supported by burgeoning research, shows significant benefits in insulin sensitivity, weight management, and overall energy levels, facilitating a deeper understanding and control over our eating habits.
- **Balanced, Mindful Eating:** Emphasizing balanced meals with adequate protein, healthy fats, and complex carbohydrates supports not just physical health but mental and emotional well-being. Mindful eating encourages us to be fully present with our food, savoring each bite and recognizing our body's hunger and fullness signals, further nurturing our good wolf.

The Role of Community in Our Nutritional Journey

The Two Wolves community is a vibrant ecosystem of support, motivation, and shared wisdom. Within this collective, every member is encouraged to share their experiences, challenges, and triumphs in navigating the nutritional aspects of the program. Whether it's seeking advice on meal planning, sharing a favorite recipe from the "Two Wolves Cookbook," or discussing strategies to overcome cravings, the community stands as a testament to the power of collective encouragement and accountability.

- **Engagement and Sharing:** The act of engaging with the community, asking questions, and sharing insights not only enriches your journey but also contributes to the communal pool of knowledge and support. This dynamic exchange keeps the spirit of the good wolf thriving within the pack.
- **The "Two Wolves Cookbook" and Nutritional Guidance:** Available for all participants, the cookbook is a treasure trove of recipes that align with the program's nutritional guidelines. It serves as a practical tool for feeding the good wolf, offering meals that are not only nutritious but also enjoyable and satisfying.

Mindfulness: The Key to Transformation

Mindfulness, the practice of being fully present and engaged in the moment, is woven throughout every aspect of the Two Wolves program. In the context of nutrition, mindfulness teaches us to be intentional about what we consume, why we consume it, and how it makes us feel. This awareness brings a deeper connection to our food, our bodies, and the choices we make, reinforcing the program's core message: the wolf we feed is the wolf that leads.

Which Wolf Are You Feeding Today?

"The one you feed is the one that leads." Each day presents a new opportunity to choose nourishment that feeds the good wolf, fostering a healthier, stronger, and more connected version of yourself. Let this be a journey of discovery, transformation, and empowerment, guided by the principles of nutrition, the support of our community, and the practice of mindfulness.

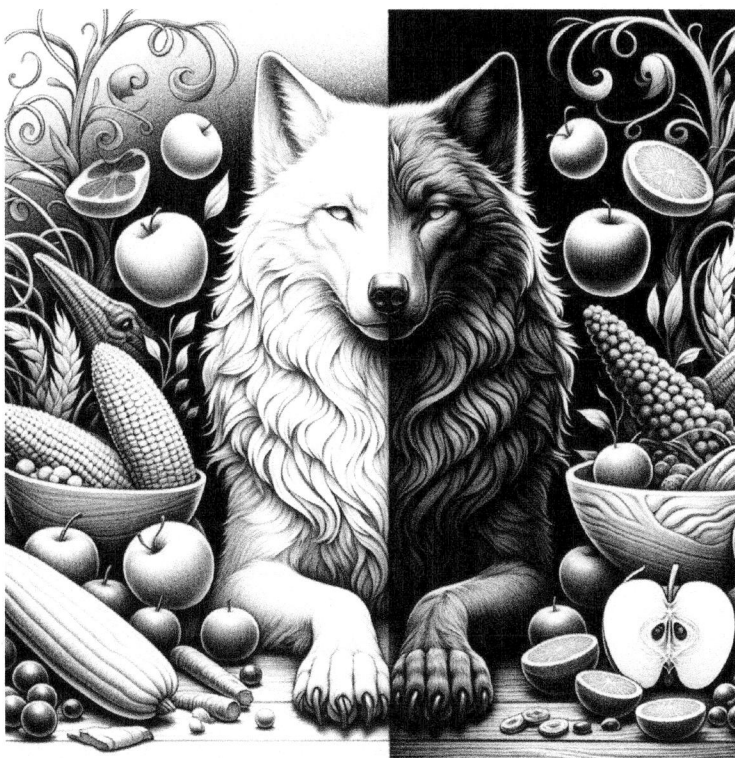

Shopping List (optional)

As you navigate the aisles of the supermarket, aiming to nourish the good wolf within, here's a basic list of foods to prioritize in your shopping cart. These selections are designed to support a well-rounded, nutritious diet that aligns with the principles of the Two Wolves program:

Proteins:

- Chicken breast: Lean and versatile for numerous recipes.
- Salmon and other fatty fish: Rich in Omega-3 fatty acids for heart health.
- Eggs: A complete protein source, perfect for any meal.
- Tofu and tempeh: Great plant-based protein options for vegetarians and vegans.
- Lean beef and turkey: For a variety of protein-rich meals.

Fruits and Vegetables:

- Leafy greens (spinach, kale, arugula): Packed with vitamins, minerals, and fiber.
- Berries (strawberries, blueberries, raspberries): High in antioxidants and low in sugar.
- Apples and bananas: Convenient, nutrient-dense snacks.
- Cruciferous vegetables (broccoli, cauliflower, Brussels sprouts): Excellent for digestion and full of nutrients.
- Sweet potatoes: A healthier carbohydrate option, rich in beta-carotene.

Whole Grains:

- Quinoa: A complete protein and great base for salads and side dishes.
- Brown rice: A versatile whole grain that pairs well with almost any meal.
- Whole wheat or whole grain pasta and bread: For when you need a pasta fix or a sandwich.

- Oats: Perfect for a hearty breakfast that keeps you full.

Healthy Fats:
- Avocados: Full of healthy fats and fiber.
- Nuts and seeds (almonds, chia seeds, flaxseeds): Great for snacking or adding a crunch to salads.
- Olive oil: A heart-healthy oil ideal for cooking and dressings.

Dairy and Dairy Alternatives:
- Greek yogurt: High in protein and probiotics.
- Almond milk or other plant-based milks: Look for unsweetened versions.
- Cheese: Opt for lower-fat varieties or plant-based alternatives.

Miscellaneous:
- Legumes (chickpeas, lentils, black beans): Fiber-rich and versatile for many dishes.
- Herbs and spices: To add flavor without the extra calories or sodium.
- Water or sparkling water: Stay hydrated and avoid sugary drinks.
- Tea, especially green tea: Offers a healthy dose of antioxidants.

When shopping, aim to fill your cart with these whole, unprocessed foods, focusing on variety and balance to ensure you're receiving all the necessary nutrients to support your journey with the Two Wolves program. The list provided above is meant as suggestions and guidance to aid in your nutritional choices, serving as a foundation upon which to build a balanced and healthful diet. It's essential to employ logic in your selections but also to choose foods that you know you can consistently enjoy and adhere to. Remember, the pillars of consistency, simplicity, and accountability are key to your success in the Two Wolves program. To further support your journey, consider posting your shopping list in the community for advice, feedback, and encouragement from fellow pack members. This not only helps refine your choices but also strengthens the communal bond, keeping you motivated and on track towards achieving your health and wellness goals.

Daily 7: Packwork

At the heart of the Two Wolves program lies a deeply structured, purposeful approach to personal transformation that transcends mere physical change, delving into the realms of mental, emotional, and spiritual growth. This holistic journey is navigated through daily engagements with educational material, reflective tracking, and journaling—an odyssey of learning that each day unfurls a new chapter and lesson on the multifaceted aspects of health, fitness, and mindfulness.

A Curriculum for Transformation:
Each day of the program is meticulously designed as a new chapter in your journey, presenting a lesson that enriches your understanding and application of the principles central to health, fitness, and mindfulness. From the science behind nutritional choices and the mechanics of effective workout routines to the practices of meditation and the art of self-reflection, the program covers a broad spectrum of subject material. This daily dose of knowledge isn't just about imparting information; it's about weaving these insights into the fabric of your daily life, making transformation an accessible reality.

Journaling: A Keystone Practice:
Central to this journey is the practice of journaling how you feel each day. This isn't a mere record-keeping exercise but a profound process of introspection and self-discovery. By documenting your emotional and mental state, you engage in a dialogue with yourself, uncovering insights about your motivations, challenges, and victories. This practice fosters a deepened self-awareness and a mindful presence in your transformation process, setting the Two Wolves program apart from any other challenge out there.

The Power of Reflection:

Taking notes and reflecting on the day's lesson allows you to crystallize your learning, transforming abstract concepts into personal wisdom. This act of reflection is crucial; it ensures that each lesson resonates with your personal journey, helping you to navigate the complexities of change with greater clarity and confidence. As Confucius once said, "Learning without thought is labor lost; thought without learning is perilous." Our program embodies this philosophy, encouraging participants to not only learn but to ponder and internalize the day's teachings.

Engagement and Community:

Moreover, this daily engagement fosters a sense of accountability and commitment, not just to the program, but more importantly, to oneself. It's a daily recommitment to your journey of growth and the goals you've set. Additionally, sharing your reflections and insights within the Two Wolves community cultivates a shared learning environment, where collective wisdom bolsters individual journeys, creating a web of support that is both inspiring and empowering.

Embracing the Journey:

Each day's chapter and lesson in the Two Wolves program are steps on a path toward holistic well-being. They are designed to challenge, inspire, and transform you, covering the expanse of health, fitness, and mindfulness in a way that is integrated and comprehensive. This journey is unique in its approach, ensuring that as you evolve physically, you are also growing mentally, emotionally, and spiritually.

The integration of daily study, reflection, and journaling is what makes the Two Wolves program profoundly impactful. It is an invitation to embark on a journey of true transformation, where every day is an opportunity to learn, to reflect, and to become a little more the person you aspire to be. This holistic approach ensures that as you nourish and train your body, you are also nurturing your mind and spirit, feeding the good wolf within and embracing the full spectrum of your potential.

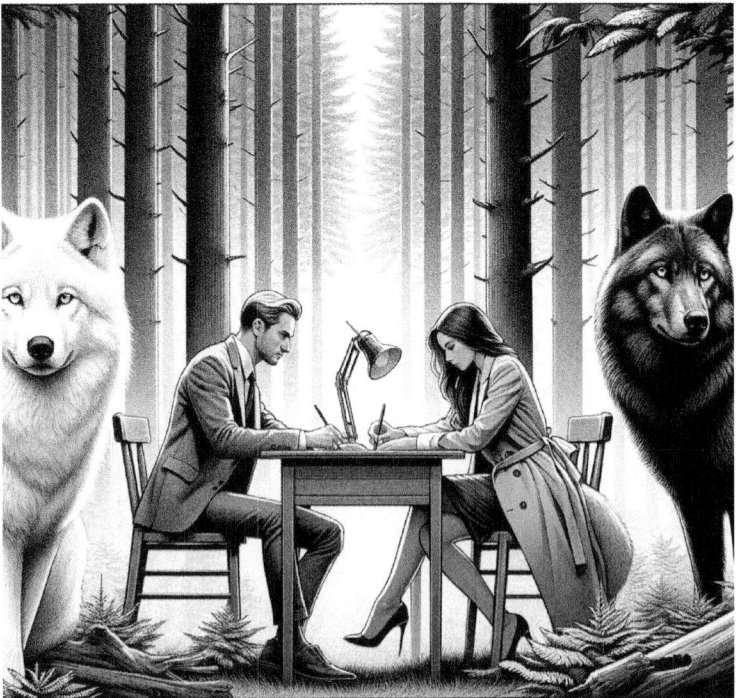

Daily 8: Supplements*

At the outset of this discussion on the role of supplements within the Two Wolves program, it's essential to underscore that their use is entirely optional. As the term itself implies, supplements are meant to complement—not substitute—the foundational pillars of your wellness journey. They can undoubtedly offer benefits, augmenting your progress towards holistic health. However, it's crucial to remember that a complete and total transformation does not hinge on their inclusion. The Two Wolves program is meticulously designed to be comprehensive and self-sufficient, requiring nothing more than dedication, the guidance provided by this book, and your commitment to growth. We stand firm in the belief that the core tenets of the program—mindful nutrition, consistent physical activity, and deep self-reflection—are potent enough to catalyze profound change.

Multivitamin: Multivitamins serve as a comprehensive source of essential vitamins and minerals, ensuring you meet your daily nutritional needs. A study published in Nutrients (2017) highlighted the role of multivitamin supplementation in filling nutritional gaps and supporting overall health, especially in populations at risk of deficiencies.

Magnesium: Magnesium is pivotal for over 300 biochemical reactions in the body, including muscle and nerve function, blood glucose control, and energy production. Research in the Journal of the American College of Nutrition (2012) suggests that magnesium supplementation can improve metabolic markers and support healthy blood pressure levels, underscoring its importance in a balanced diet.

*optional

Fish Oil (Omega-3 Fatty Acids): Omega-3 fatty acids, particularly EPA and DHA found in fish oil, are essential for brain health and reducing inflammation. A meta-analysis in JAMA Cardiology (2017) concluded that omega-3 supplementation is associated with a reduced risk of heart-related deaths, highlighting its cardiovascular benefits.

Vitamin D: Vitamin D plays a crucial role in bone health, immune function, and reducing inflammation. Given that many people have limited sun exposure, supplementation can be necessary to achieve adequate levels. According to the American Journal of Clinical Nutrition (2012), vitamin D supplementation has been shown to improve bone health and reduce the risk of falls in older adults.

Probiotics: Probiotics support gut health by maintaining a healthy balance of gut flora, which can positively impact digestion and the immune system. A review in Nutrients (2016) found that probiotic supplementation could enhance digestive health and may contribute to improved mental health through the gut-brain axis.

Green Powder (Super Greens): Super greens powders are made from a blend of nutrient-dense plants and offer a convenient way to increase your intake of vitamins, minerals, and antioxidants. While direct studies on green powders are limited, research supports the health benefits of consuming a diet rich in fruits and vegetables, as indicated in a review in The Lancet (2017), which suggests such diets can lower the risk of heart disease, stroke, and certain cancers.

It's important to note that while supplements can provide additional nutritional support, they should not replace a balanced diet and healthy lifestyle. Always consult with a healthcare professional before starting any new supplement regimen, especially if you have existing health conditions or are taking medications. The Two Wolves program emphasizes a holistic approach to wellness, with or without supplementation, focusing on nourishing the body, cultivating the mind, and fostering spiritual growth through consistent, mindful practices.

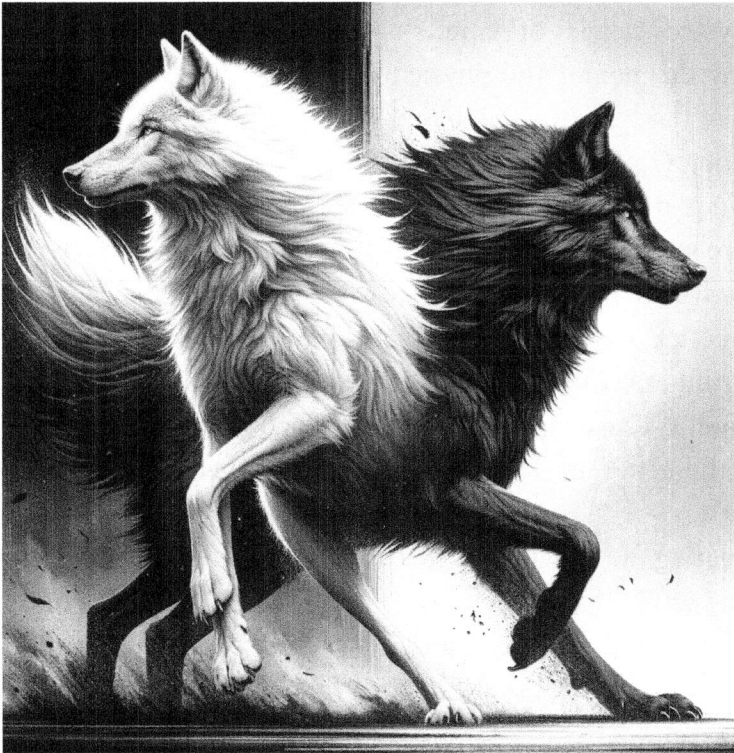

Daily 9: Sleep

Sleep stands as a pillar of health within the Two Wolves program, vital for harmonizing our physical, mental, and emotional states. Embracing the wisdom of Benjamin Franklin, who noted, "Early to bed and early to rise, makes a man healthy, wealthy, and wise," we recognize the importance of securing 7-9 hours of restorative sleep each night. This practice isn't merely about quantity but also the quality of sleep, crucial for the body's restorative processes like tissue repair, protein synthesis, and memory consolidation.

The Science of Sleep:
Research underscores the critical role sleep plays in our well-being. Disruptions in sleep patterns have been linked to various health issues, from heart disease and diabetes to obesity and cognitive impairments. As Shakespeare elegantly put it, "Sleep that knits up the raveled sleave of care..."—sleep is indeed our daily reset, mending the mental and physical exertions of the day.

Promoting Optimal Sleep:
Achieving quality sleep requires both commitment and strategy. Here are science-backed methods to enhance your sleep hygiene:
- **Consistent Sleep Routine:** Establishing a regular bedtime and wake-up schedule aligns with your body's natural circadian rhythm, promoting better sleep quality.
- **Mindful Consumption:** Limit caffeine and stimulants, especially in the latter part of the day, to avoid disrupting your sleep cycle.
- **Creating a Sanctuary:** Ensure your sleeping environment is conducive to rest—quiet, dark, and at a comfortable temperature. As Da Vinci observed, "*A well-spent day brings happy sleep,*" so too does a well-prepared bedroom invite restful slumber.

- **Wind-Down Rituals:** Engage in calming activities before bed, such as deep breathing, meditation, or reading. These practices can signal to your body that it's time to wind down, easing the transition into sleep.

Patience and Consistency:
Adopting these sleep-promoting habits may not yield immediate results, but with consistency, improvements will manifest. As with any change, the body and mind need time to adjust. Embrace this process with patience and persistence, knowing that each night's effort contributes to the greater goal of enhanced well-being.

Sleep's Place in Holistic Health:
Incorporating these sleep practices into your daily routine is more than an act of self-care—it's a foundational element of the holistic approach championed by the Two Wolves program. Quality sleep enriches our lives, empowering us to face each day with renewed vigor, clarity, and emotional balance.

Remember, the journey to better sleep and, by extension, to improved health and wellness, is a gradual process that unfolds with daily commitment. By nurturing our sleep, we nurture our entire being, laying the foundation for a life lived in harmony with our body's natural rhythms and needs.

Daily 10: Progress Tracking

Incorporating daily progress photos into your fitness journey stands as a transformative strategy within the Two Wolves program, offering a clear, visual chronicle of your physical evolution. This practice isn't merely about capturing images; it's a scientific and motivational approach to tracking and celebrating the changes your body undergoes, providing both inspiration and insight into your personal growth.

The Science of Visualization:
Research in the field of sports psychology emphasizes the power of visualization in achieving fitness goals. Seeing tangible evidence of your progress can significantly boost your motivation, reinforcing your commitment to the program. It acts as a visual affirmation of your hard work, often translating into heightened self-confidence and a renewed vigor to pursue your goals.

Identifying Areas for Improvement:
Beyond motivation, progress photos serve as an invaluable tool for personal assessment. By systematically analyzing photos from various angles and over intervals, you're equipped to discern which aspects of your fitness regimen are yielding results and which areas might require more focused effort. This objective analysis can guide necessary adjustments in your workout or nutrition plans, fostering more balanced and comprehensive development.

Tips for Consistent and Effective Progress Photos:
- Consistency in Conditions: Ensure photos are taken under similar lighting and at the same time of day to maintain consistency. This accuracy is crucial for reliable comparison over time.

- **Uniformity in Appearance:** Opt for consistent attire and poses in each photo. This standardization removes variables, making subtle changes more noticeable.
- **Comprehensive Angles:** Capture front, back, and side views with each session. Viewing your progress from multiple perspectives offers a fuller picture of your physical transformation.
- **Patience and Persistence:** Transformation is a gradual process. While daily changes might be subtle, the cumulative effect over time can be profound. Trust in the journey and the process laid out by the Two Wolves program.

Capturing Your Journey:
To effectively track your journey, consider these practical steps:
- **Use the Same Camera:** Consistency in equipment eliminates variations in image quality and framing.
- **Optimal Lighting:** Seek out natural light or a well-lit setting to ensure clarity and detail in your photos.
- **Standardized Attire and Position:** Consistent clothing and poses across your photos make comparisons more straightforward and meaningful.
- **Routine Timing:** Taking photos at a regular time each day establishes a reliable baseline for tracking changes.

Remember, the purpose of progress photos is to document and celebrate your journey, not to critique. Each photo is a milestone in your path to wellness, a testament to your dedication and hard work. While sharing these milestones within the community can be a source of support and encouragement, know that disclosure is entirely at your discretion. The Two Wolves program champions building confidence at your own pace, acknowledging that each individual's journey is unique. Embrace this practice as a powerful ally in your transformation, understanding that with consistency and patience, the rewards will unfold.

Heart Rate Zones

XII

Understanding your heart rate zones is a valuable aspect of tailoring your workout's intensity to your body's responses, enhancing the efficiency of your exercise regimen. While the latest gadgets like heart rate monitors and fitness trackers offer precise insights into your heart rate zones, it's essential to recognize that these tools are not prerequisites for effective workout management. Modern smartphones and smartwatches often come equipped with features that facilitate heart rate tracking, making this technology more accessible than ever.

The Talk Test: A Simple Yet Effective Method
A straightforward alternative to technology-based monitoring is the talk test. This method involves assessing your ability to converse during exercise. If you can comfortably engage in a conversation, you're likely operating within the fat-burning zone, which is generally 60-70% of your maximum heart rate. This zone signifies that your body is utilizing fat as its primary energy source. However, maximum heart rate varies individually, emphasizing the benefit of consulting with a fitness professional to personalize your heart rate zones.

Adaptation in the Cub Program
In the initial stages of the Two Wolves program, particularly at the Cub level, the emphasis lies on fostering a habit of regular physical activity that aligns with your enjoyment and comfort. The intricacies of heart rate zones, while informative, are not the focal point at this juncture. As you ascend through the program's levels, reaching Delta and beyond, we delve into the strategic application of heart rate zones to maximize the effectiveness of your workouts, tapping into the primal energy of your "wolf heart."

The Path to Fitness Mastery

Embarking on your fitness journey is a process marked by gradual improvement and learning. Familiarizing yourself with the concept of heart rate zones contributes to a more nuanced understanding of your physical endeavors, enabling you to tailor the intensity of your exercises thoughtfully. This knowledge empowers you to make well-informed choices that complement your comprehensive fitness objectives.

As you navigate through your journey, remember that progress is measured in steady steps forward, fueled by curiosity and a deep connection to your body's signals. With or without advanced tracking equipment, your commitment to moving, exploring, and tuning in to your heart's rhythm carves the path to achieving your fitness aspirations. Stay dedicated, remain inquisitive, and trust in the strength and resilience of your heart.

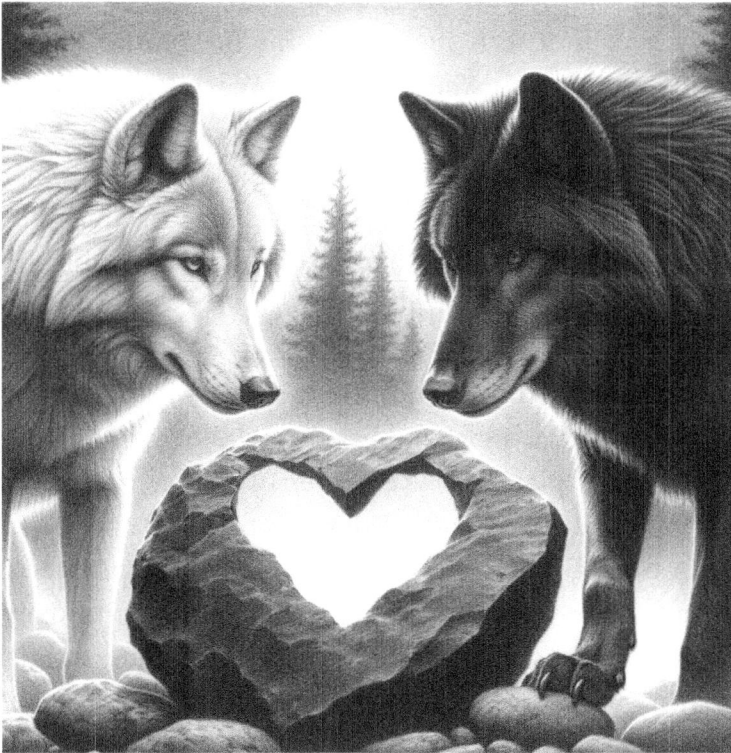

Own your morning
Own your day
XIII

The way we usher in the day has a profound impact on the tapestry of our daily experiences. Mastering the morning is akin to setting the stage for a play; each action and decision contributes to the narrative of success, productivity, and well-being. This chapter draws upon the wisdom of modern thought leaders and timeless classical quotes to inspire and guide you toward seizing control of your mornings and, by extension, your life.

The Ritual of Order and Achievement

Beginning each day by making your bed is a simple yet transformative habit. This act is championed by Admiral William H. McRaven, who asserts in Make Your Bed: Little Things That Can Change Your Life...And Maybe the World, "*If you make your bed every morning, you will have accomplished the first task of the day.*" This task, though small, sets a tone of accomplishment and order, serving as a metaphor for taking charge of your life. It's a physical manifestation of the inner discipline and organization you aim to apply throughout your day.

Guidance Through Intentional Planning

The significance of a morning checklist cannot be overstated. As Charles Duhigg explains in The Power of Habit, routines are the backbone of productive habits. Your cub program checklist acts as a roadmap through your day, with each ticked box symbolizing a step closer to your goals. This methodical approach to daily tasks fosters a satisfying sense of progress, echoing the sentiments of Seneca: "*It is not that we have so little time but that we lose so much. ... The life we receive is not short but we make it so; we are not ill-provided but use what we have wastefully.*"

Hydration as a Keystone Habit

The importance of starting your day with water is highlighted by the physiological need to hydrate after hours of sleep. James Clear, in Atomic Habits, articulates the power of keystone habits in catalyzing widespread changes in our lives. Morning hydration kickstarts your metabolism, cleanses your system, and sets a precedent for making health-conscious decisions throughout the day. This aligns with the principle that *"Small changes often will compound into remarkable results over time."*

The Value of a Conscious Awakening

The act of waking up immediately upon your alarm sounding is a commitment to starting your day with purpose. As Robin Sharma argues in The 5 AM Club, mastering your morning begins with the victory of rising early, engaging in activities that nurture your mind, body, and spirit. Resisting the snooze button is more than a physical act—it's a declaration that you are ready and willing to greet the day with enthusiasm and energy.

Incorporating Movement and Mindfulness

Incorporating physical activity into your morning routine is essential for awakening both the body and mind. As Thoreau noted, *"An early-morning walk is a blessing for the whole day."* Whether it's yoga, a brisk walk, or a workout session, morning exercise primes you for the day ahead, enhancing focus, mood, and physical stamina.

The Symphony of the Morning

Mastering the morning is about more than the sum of its parts; it's about creating a symphony of habits that resonate with the rhythm of success and well-being. Each element—from making your bed to embracing the first light of day with activity and intention—plays a crucial role in this daily overture. Drawing on the insights of modern authors and the timeless wisdom encapsulated in classical quotes, this chapter serves as a beacon, guiding you towards embracing each morning not just as the start of a new day, but as the dawn of infinite possibilities.

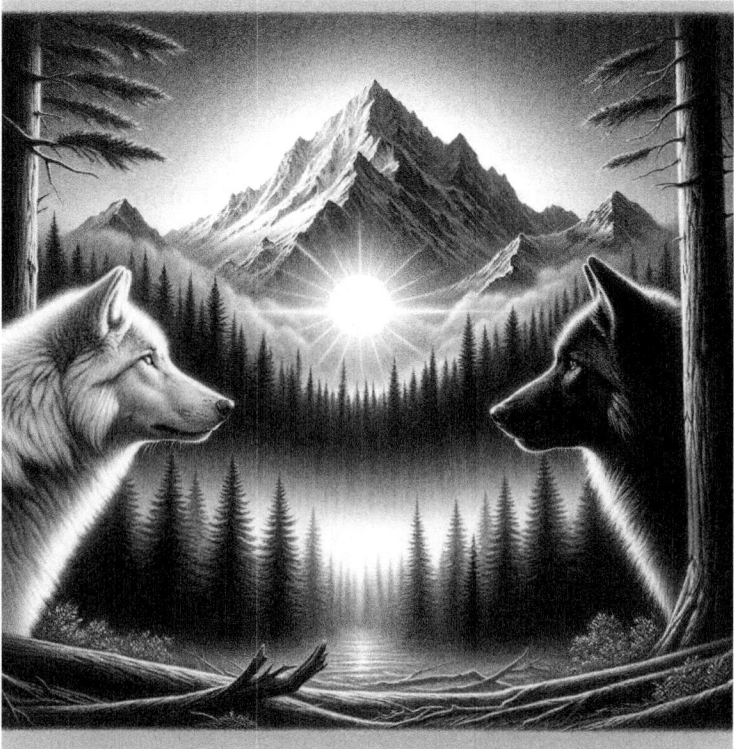

Journaling the Journey

XIV

The potency of the written word transcends its simplicity, emerging as a profound conduit for transformation. Engaging with pen and paper unlocks a realm of self-exploration and heightened awareness, allowing us to articulate the silent whispers of our hearts and minds. This act of inscription, central to the "Writing it Down" exercise, stands as a cornerstone of the Two Wolves program, facilitating a journey into the depths of our being.

Activating the Mind's Eye

Engaging in the practice of writing does more than capture thoughts—it enlivens a part of the brain known as the Reticular Activating System (RAS). The RAS acts as a sentinel, sifting through the multitude of stimuli we encounter, and honing our focus on what truly matters. Writing, therefore, is not merely a record-keeping exercise but a dynamic process of engagement, enabling us to clarify and process our inner experiences, emotions, and aspirations.

Journaling: A Scientifically Backed Practice

The benefits of journaling are well-documented across numerous studies, highlighting its ability to mitigate stress, enhance mood, and fortify the immune system. These effects underscore journaling's role in not only navigating but also flourishing amidst life's complexities.

Dr. Joe Dispenza champions the transformative potential of writing in "Breaking the Habit of Being Yourself," where he delves into how documenting our ambitions and reflections can rewire the subconscious mind. This act of setting intentions and articulating visions serves as a beacon, guiding our thoughts and energies towards the essence of what we seek to manifest in our lives.

A Tool for Unveiling the Inner Wolf
Within the tapestry of the Two Wolves program, journaling emerges as a vital instrument for introspection and growth. This practice illuminates the path to recognizing and embracing our inner wolf—a symbol of courage, resilience, and hope. Through reflective writing, we unearth the barriers to our progress, allowing us to confront and navigate through them with newfound perspective and strength.

Embrace the Power of Your Words
As you embark on this journey of journaling, let each word you write be a step towards self-discovery and empowerment. Reflect on your strides in the program, articulate your dreams, and confront your fears. Remember, your narrative holds the power to transform, to heal, and to reveal the boundless potential that resides within.

In penning down your story, you not only chronicle your journey but also lay the foundation for a profound metamorphosis. Your words are the architects of your destiny, the keys to unlocking your true self, and the catalysts for embodying the spirit of the Two Wolves program. Let the ink flow, and watch as the pages of your life unfold into a masterpiece of personal triumph and enlightenment.

The Double Up

XV

In the whirlwind of our daily lives, where time is a precious commodity, the concept of task doubling emerges as a revolutionary strategy to enhance productivity. Task doubling, or multitasking with purpose, allows us to weave together various activities, maximizing our efficiency and enriching our lives with a tapestry of accomplishments.

Synergizing Fitness with Learning

Embark on the journey of physical and mental growth by merging exercise with intellectual or spiritual enrichment. Imagine absorbing the wisdom of a motivational audiobook or the tranquility of a guided meditation as you stride through your morning jog or yoga session. This fusion not only amplifies the benefits to your physical well-being but also elevates your mental clarity and emotional balance, creating a holistic harmony between body and mind.

Mindfulness in Motion

Transform routine chores into moments of zen by infusing them with mindfulness practices. As you engage in the simplicity of tasks like washing dishes or organizing your space, focus deeply on your breath or the sensations of the activity. This approach turns mundane tasks into meditative practices, fostering a sense of presence and calmness amidst the day's hustle.

Learning on the Go

Convert your commute into a mobile classroom by delving into a new skill or language through podcasts or audiobooks.

Whether you're navigating through traffic or aboard public transport, this practice turns idle time into a valuable learning experience, broadening your horizons and sparking new interests with each mile.

Combining Connection with Activity

Redefine quality time with loved ones by integrating it with physical activities. Plan outings that encourage movement, such as hiking, biking, or a friendly game of sports. These shared experiences not only fortify personal bonds but also promote health and well-being, enriching your relationships with the joy of shared achievements.

Strategies for Seamless Task Doubling

To seamlessly integrate task doubling into your routine, consider the following tips:

- **Prioritize Compatibility:** Choose tasks that naturally complement each other, ensuring one activity doesn't detract from the quality or focus of the other.
- **Set Clear Goals:** Define what you wish to achieve with each combined activity to maintain direction and purpose.
- **Embrace Flexibility:** Be open to adjusting your combinations based on what works best for your lifestyle and objectives.
- **Reflect on Outcomes:** Periodically assess the effectiveness of your task doubling strategies, making adjustments as needed to optimize your productivity and satisfaction.

Embracing Efficiency

Task doubling is more than a productivity hack; it's a lifestyle choice that champions the efficient use of time, enabling us to lead richer, more balanced lives. By thoughtfully pairing activities, we unlock the potential to achieve more, experience more, and ultimately, become more. In the words of Henry David Thoreau, *"It's not enough to be busy; so are the ants. The question is: what are we busy about?"* Let task doubling be your answer, crafting a life that's as productive as it is purposeful.

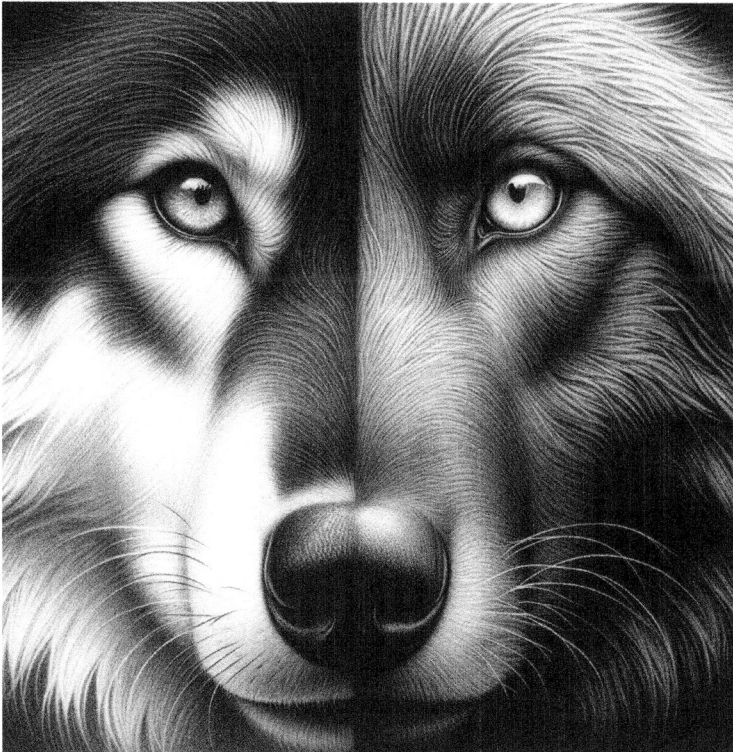

The Pack

XVI

Within the human spirit lies a profound yearning for connection and community—a fundamental need to belong and thrive alongside others. This intrinsic social nature is especially pronounced on the path to self-improvement, where the quest for health and wellness often feels like an insurmountable expedition. Yet, this journey is transformed from a solitary trek into a communal voyage with the support and camaraderie of a dedicated group.

Embracing the Pack in the Two Wolves Program
Joining the Two Wolves program immerses you in a pack of individuals who share your aspirations for health and personal betterment. This community acts as a beacon of encouragement, understanding, and accountability, guiding you through the intricacies of your wellness journey. It's more than a collection of individuals; it's a sanctum of shared experiences, challenges, and triumphs.

The Strength of Belonging
At the core of the pack's essence is the profound sense of belonging it offers. Aristotle once said, "The whole is greater than the sum of its parts," a sentiment that resonates deeply within the dynamics of the pack. This belonging fuels your motivation and fortifies your commitment, empowering you to persevere towards your goals with renewed vigor.

Accountability and Shared Endeavors
The pack not only provides companionship but also holds you accountable, ensuring you remain steadfast on your path. This collective endeavor amplifies your capacity to succeed, allowing you to draw upon the group's energy and wisdom.

Sharing both victories and setbacks with the pack not only lightens the burden but also multiplies the joy, fostering a nurturing environment of guidance and mutual support.

Survival and Thriving Together

Mirroring the natural world, where wolves band together for survival, the pack in the Two Wolves program symbolizes our collective strength and resilience. Together, you navigate challenges, safeguarding each other's progress and nurturing the group's well-being. This solidarity is the cornerstone of overcoming obstacles and celebrating successes as a unified entity.

A Sanctuary of Growth and Learning

The pack is more than just a support system; it's a sacred space for authenticity, shared learning, and mutual growth. It's a haven built on the pillars of trust, respect, and unwavering support. Within this community, you're not just embarking on a personal transformation; you're contributing to a larger movement of collective empowerment.

Becoming Part of Something Greater

Joining the pack transcends individual accomplishment, inviting you into a fellowship of collective aspiration and achievement. It's an empowering journey where each member's progress uplifts the entire group, creating a powerful force of communal wellbeing and transformation.

In the Two Wolves program, the pack is your ally, your mentor, and your cheerleader, embodying the program's essence and propelling you towards realizing the fullest potential of your health and wellness goals. Together, as a pack, the journey towards self-improvement becomes not only attainable but an adventure of shared destiny and collective triumph.

Embarking on this transformative path is just a step away. By joining the pack through the link provided, you unlock the door to a community brimming with camaraderie, support, and mutual growth. This portal is not merely a means to enroll in the Two Wolves program but a bridge to a realm where each individual's journey is amplified by the collective strength and wisdom of the group. Here, within the pack, you find more than just members; you discover allies, mentors, and friends all united by a common goal of wellness and self-discovery.

Join the Pack [links at the back of the book]

This link is your invitation to become part of a community that values each member's progress as a collective victory. It's a step towards not just achieving your personal health and wellness goals but also contributing to a movement of positive transformation that extends beyond individual boundaries. By joining the pack, you embrace a role in a story much larger than your own—a narrative of empowerment, resilience, and shared success.

Welcome to the pack, where together, we embark on a journey of transformation, navigating the path of wellness with the support and strength of a community that believes in the power of unity and the spirit of collective achievement.

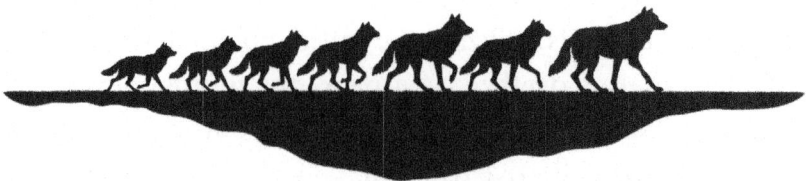

Pre-Pack-Initiation

XVII

Embarking on the Two Wolves program, you're about to transform more than just your physical appearance; you're setting the stage for a profound personal evolution. Success in this transformative journey hinges on strategic preparation, ensuring that every element of your daily routine aligns with your goals. From nourishing your body with carefully selected meals to embracing the discipline of exercise, the initial steps you take are pivotal in sculpting the path to success.

Crafting Your Nutritional Compass

Incorporating an 8-hour eating window into your daily schedule is a cornerstone of the Two Wolves program, promoting a mindful approach to nutrition while aligning with intermittent fasting principles. Begin by designing a meal plan that not only satisfies your nutritional needs but also fits seamlessly into this eating window. Plan nutrient-dense, balanced meals for breakfast, lunch, and dinner that will keep you energized and satiated throughout your active hours. Preparing a grocery list tailored to these meals will streamline your shopping process, making healthy choices the default rather than the exception.

Establishing Your Physical Baseline

Before you dive into the heart of the program, it's crucial to understand where you stand physically. The "Wolf Tracker" assessments provide a clear picture of your starting point. Perform initial tests—such as measuring the length of time you can hold a plank and the number of jumping jacks you can complete in one minute—to set your baseline metrics. These figures are not just numbers; they're the starting line of your race towards transformation, offering a tangible means to measure your progress.

A Visual Pledge to Your Future Self

Taking 'before' photos is more than a formality; it's a commitment to the journey you're about to undertake. Approach this task with the seriousness it deserves—these images mark the beginning of your transformation. Wearing attire that accurately reflects your current physical state, capture shots from various angles to fully document your starting point. These photos will serve not just as a reminder of where you began but as a testament to how far you've come, once you cross the finish line of this program.

Solidifying Bonds Within the Pack

The power of the pack lies not only in shared goals but in the collective journey towards achieving them. Introducing yourself to this community is the first step in building connections that will support, challenge, and inspire you throughout the program. Share your aspirations, learn from others' experiences, and offer your encouragement. This network of peers becomes a source of strength, propelling you forward even on the toughest days.

Embracing the Journey Ahead

As you stand on the precipice of change, remember that the success of your journey through the Two Wolves program begins with meticulous preparation. By tailoring your nutrition to fit an 8-hour eating window, assessing your physical capabilities, documenting your starting point, and connecting with your pack, you're not just preparing for a fitness program; you're laying the foundation for a life-altering journey. With every planned meal, every baseline test, and every new connection, you're one step closer to unveiling the strongest, healthiest version of yourself. Let's begin.

Equipment List

XVIII

The Two Wolves program celebrates simplicity and accessibility, emphasizing that transformation doesn't require complexity or high-tech equipment. To set you on the path to success, here are a few basic items that can enhance your experience:

- **Comfortable Workout Attire:** Select clothes that offer comfort and flexibility. Whether it's yoga pants, running shorts, or breathable tees, the right outfit can make your workout more enjoyable and effective.
- **Supportive Athletic Shoes:** The foundation of many exercises, a reliable pair of athletic shoes, is crucial. Look for footwear that provides stability and comfort, tailored to your activity of choice.
- **Hydration Companion:** A durable water bottle is your ally in maintaining hydration throughout your fitness endeavors. Opt for a refillable bottle to keep water on hand, ensuring you stay hydrated before, during, and after workouts.
- **Yoga Mat:** For those floor exercises and stretches, a yoga mat offers a supportive surface, cushioning your body and enhancing your exercise experience.
- **Smartwatch (Optional):** While not essential for the Cub program, a basic fitness tracker can be a useful tool for monitoring activity levels and progress. There are affordable options available that cover the essentials without overwhelming you with unnecessary features.
- **Step-Tracking App:** Harness the power of technology with a free step-tracking app, such as StepsApp, to monitor your daily movements. These apps motivate you to reach your daily step goals and provide insights into your activity patterns.

- **Sleep Tracking App:** Quality rest is just as important as active workouts. Utilize a sleep-tracking app like Sleep Cycle to analyze your sleep patterns and optimize your rest for maximum recovery and performance.

Getting Started with What You Have

It's important to remember that these items are merely tools to aid your journey. The heart of the Two Wolves program lies in your commitment, consistency, and drive to embrace healthier habits. Begin with whatever resources you currently have at your disposal and gradually build your toolkit as you progress. Most importantly, each step you take, whether equipped with the basics or fully kitted out, moves you closer to your wellness goals.

Regarding app subscriptions, many offer valuable features without the need for premium upgrades. Simply bypass any payment prompts by selecting 'ignore' or tapping the 'X', usually found in the top right corner. This way, you can enjoy the benefits of these tools without incurring extra costs.

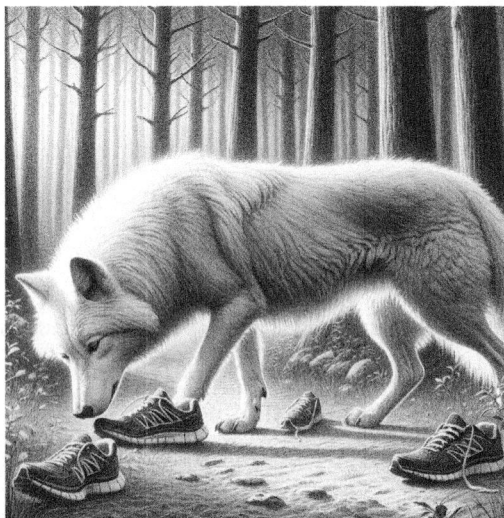

Expectations

XIX

As you embark on the transformative odyssey with the Two Wolves program, navigating the sea of expectations becomes an essential skill. Expectations, much like the wind, have the power to propel us forward with hope and ambition or capsize our spirits with the weight of disappointment. Aristotle once remarked, *"Knowing yourself is the beginning of all wisdom,"* a sentiment that underscores the importance of setting expectations that are rooted in self-awareness and tailored to our individual journeys.

Beyond Weight Loss: Embracing a Comprehensive Wellness Philosophy

At the heart of the Two Wolves program lies a holistic approach that seeks to harmonize the mind and body. Our mission extends beyond the superficial goal of weight loss, focusing instead on fostering a robust mindset and a thriving physical state. This comprehensive approach is supported by research, such as a study in the Journal of Health Psychology which finds that individuals who adopt a holistic view of health, integrating mental and physical wellness, are more likely to sustain long-term health improvements.

Understanding the Dynamics of Weight Management

Embarking on a weight loss journey without recognizing its inherent complexities can set the stage for frustration. It's vital to acknowledge that weight management is influenced by a multitude of factors, including genetics, metabolism, and lifestyle choices. A study published in Obesity Reviews highlights the non-linear nature of weight loss, emphasizing the importance of setting realistic expectations and focusing on overall health rather than short-term scale victories.

Redefining Progress: Beyond the Scale

True progress in your wellness journey manifests in myriad forms, from enhanced mental clarity and emotional resilience to increased physical strength and stamina. The American Journal of Public Health suggests that improvements in physical fitness and mental well-being are significant predictors of long-term health outcomes, far surpassing the singular metric of weight. These facets of progress, often overlooked, are where the transformative power of the Two Wolves program truly shines.

Cultivating Patience and Celebrating Milestones

In the pursuit of wellness, patience is not merely a virtue but a necessity. As Henry David Thoreau wisely noted, *"Good things come to those who wait, but better things come to those who go out and get them."* This proactive patience involves celebrating each step forward, no matter how small, and recognizing the inherent value in the journey itself.

Scientific Insights and Inspirational Wisdom

Incorporating insights from behavioral science, such as those found in Psychological Science, which demonstrates the motivational power of celebrating small victories, can further enrich your journey. These findings echo the timeless wisdom of Marcus Aurelius, who advised, *"The impediment to action advances action. What stands in the way becomes the way."* In embracing every challenge as an opportunity for growth, you align more closely with your goals.

Embracing the Two Wolves Philosophy

As you venture through the Two Wolves program, armed with knowledge, patience, and a balanced set of expectations, you embark on a journey of profound transformation. This path is not defined by the immediacy of results but by the depth of your experiences and the breadth of your personal growth. In aligning your expectations with the principles of holistic wellness, supported by both science and timeless wisdom, you pave the way for a journey that transcends physical achievements, leading instead to a life of balance, health, and fulfilment.

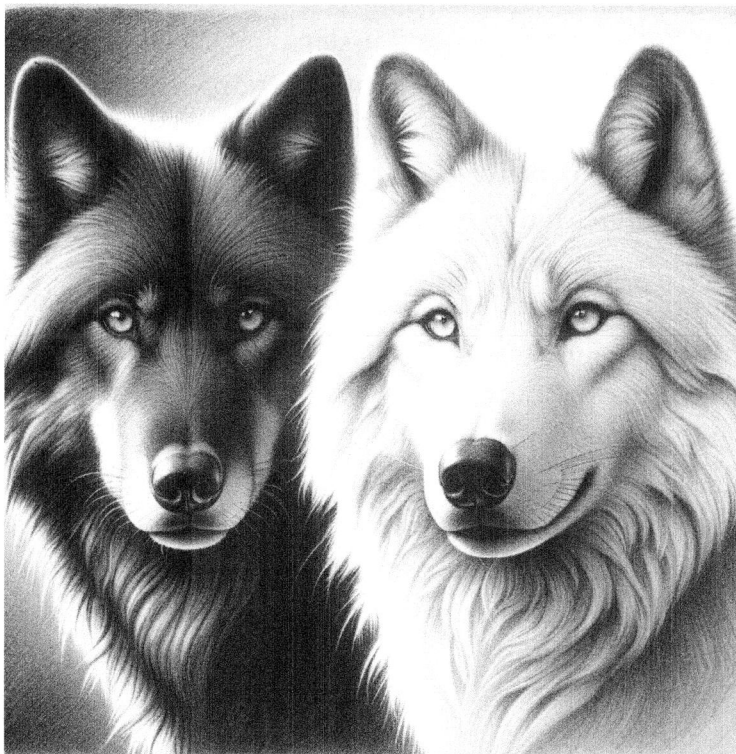

What if I fail?

XX

The quest for self-improvement and the pursuit of our goals are endeavors marked by their challenges and unforeseen hurdles. The path we embark upon is seldom straightforward; it is rife with obstacles that test our resolve and may cause us to falter. Encountering setbacks or failing to meet our own standards can lead to moments of self-doubt and disillusionment. Yet, it is within these moments of apparent failure that the seeds of growth and resilience are sown.

The Nature of Setbacks in the Two Wolves Program
The Two Wolves program is predicated on the understanding that personal growth is an intricate journey, characterized not by perfection but by perseverance. Missteps and deviations from the path are not indicators of defeat but rather opportunities for learning and self-reflection. Should you miss a day or find yourself not meeting your objectives, it's crucial to view these instances not as terminal failures but as moments ripe for growth.

Consequences as Catalysts for Growth
Within the program, missing a step or deviating from your goals triggers certain consequences, designed not as punitive measures but as mechanisms for accountability and reflection. These consequences are crafted to reinforce your commitment to your journey and to encourage a deeper engagement with your goals. They serve as reminders that every action—or inaction—carries weight, compelling us to approach our objectives with renewed focus and determination.

The Power of Community Support

At the core of the Two Wolves program is a community built on empathy, understanding, and mutual support. Within this community, every member is recognized as a fellow traveler on the path to self-discovery and improvement. Together, we share our experiences, bolstering each other through encouragement and collective wisdom. This network of support ensures that no one is left to navigate their setbacks alone; instead, we uplift and propel each other forward, transforming challenges into stepping stones for progress.

Reframing Failure as a Source of Strength

Adopting a perspective that views setbacks as vital components of the growth process allows us to emerge from challenges with enhanced resilience and wisdom. Dr. Brene Brown eloquently captures this sentiment, asserting that "*Vulnerability is not weakness; it's our greatest measure of courage.*" To err and falter is human; to acknowledge, learn from, and rise above our mistakes is to harness our inherent strength and courage.

Moving Forward with Courage and Clarity

If you find yourself facing setbacks, let this not dampen your spirit but rather fuel your resolve to persevere. Embrace the lessons borne from these experiences, allowing them to illuminate your path as you continue your journey with purpose and passion. The Two Wolves program is not merely a route to self-improvement but a voyage towards cultivating resilience, understanding, and an unwavering commitment to growth.

Together, as a community and as individuals dedicated to becoming our best selves, we embrace the ebbs and flows of our journeys. We recognize that each step back is an opportunity for a leap forward, forging paths that are all the more meaningful for the challenges we overcome.

Consequences

XXI

Navigating the path laid out by the Two Wolves program introduces us to a crucial aspect of our journey: the balance between commitment and accountability. It's here we encounter the concept of consequences—not as measures of punishment or shame but as tools for self-reflection and growth. These consequences are designed to fortify our resolve, demonstrating our dedication to the pack and to ourselves. They remind us that, while we strive for progress, accountability is key to maintaining our trajectory towards our goals.

When moments arise where we might not meet the expectations we set for ourselves—whether it's missing the mark on our 10k steps, eating outside our designated window, skipping a Wolf Workout, or indulging in alcohol—the program encourages a culture of honesty and self-discipline. Remember, straying from the path only offers us a chance to show strength in our commitment to getting back on track.

Selecting Your Consequence: A Personal Commitment
As you embark on this journey, you'll select a consequence that resonates most profoundly with you, ensuring it acts as a significant motivator to adhere to your commitments. This self-administered consequence is a testament to your integrity and determination. By embracing this system, you reaffirm your commitment not only to the program but to your personal evolution.

Consequence 1: The Path of Extra Effort [Physical] Should you find yourself needing to invoke this consequence, commit to either an additional 5,000 steps the following day or an extra set of the Wolf Workout.

This physical testament of your dedication will be shared with the pack, serving as both a personal and public acknowledgment of your resolve to push forward.

Consequence 2: Giving Back [Charitable] Choosing this consequence means committing to a charitable act, either through a donation to a local charity or by engaging in an environmental cleanup, collecting 100 pieces of litter. Documenting and sharing this act with the pack not only holds you accountable but also spreads positivity and community spirit.

Consequence 3: Embracing Abstinence This consequence involves abstaining from a chosen comfort or technology for 24 hours—be it your phone, TV, or any form of digital entertainment. This period of abstinence, followed by a reflection shared with the pack, is a powerful reminder of the importance of focus and the value of disconnecting to reconnect with our goals.

Incorporating Consequences: A Journey of Growth
As you integrate these consequences into your journey, view them not as burdens but as opportunities for growth and self-improvement. They are not penalties but pledges of perseverance, each one a step towards deeper self-awareness and stronger commitment to your path.

In the realm of the Two Wolves program, honesty, accountability, and community support are the pillars upon which we build our success. By openly declaring any missteps and embracing the consequences, you not only demonstrate your commitment to the pack but also strengthen your resolve to emerge stronger, more disciplined, and closer to achieving your goals. Remember, in the pursuit of transformation, every challenge overcome is a victory in itself.

FAQs

XXII

What types of workouts will be included in the program?
At the Cub level, we focus on callisthenic exercises, which are
bodyweight exercises that improve strength, endurance, and
flexibility. These exercises include variations of push-ups, squats,
leg-ups, planks, and step-ups. We also incorporate a 10,000-step
steady-state goal. That's it. Easy yes?!

Is the program suitable for beginners or only experienced individuals?
The Two Wolves program is suitable for individuals of all fitness
levels, including beginners. Our program is designed to gradually
increase in intensity as you progress, allowing you to build strength
and stamina over time. Our core goal is a functional connection
between the wellness of your mind which translates to external
physical results. So no matter your level of fitness, it always starts
with the wolf you feed.

**How long does each workout last? How much time will I need to
spend on this?**
Each callisthenic workout in the program will typically last around
15-20 minutes, and the recommended daily step count of 10,000
steps can be achieved throughout the day with short walks or more
structured exercise sessions. The exact time required will depend on
your fitness level and schedule, but the program is designed to be
flexible and easily adaptable to your lifestyle. In short, expect to
spend around 2 hours of your day focusing on this program.

Will I receive a nutrition plan as part of the program?
We do not offer a specific nutrition plan as part of the program.
However, we do provide some nutrition guidelines to help you

optimize your nutrition and fuel your body for optimal performance. Additionally, we offer a recipe book with 100 nutritious and delicious recipes available for purchase at a discounted price of USD$9.99. These recipes have been carefully curated to support your health and fitness goals while also satisfying your taste buds. [link at the back of the book]

Can I do the workouts at home or will I need to go to a gym?
Yes, all of the workouts in the program are designed to be done at home with little to no equipment required. The callisthenic exercises can be done with just your body weight, and the walking can be done outdoors or indoors on a treadmill. So, you can easily do the workouts from the comfort of your own home without needing to go to a gym.

What equipment will I need for the program?
As the program focuses on bodyweight exercises, no equipment is required. However, it is recommended to have a yoga mat or some padding for floor exercises, and a water bottle to stay hydrated during workouts.

How long is the program?
The initial program is 30 days, designed to establish a strong foundation of healthy habits and to kickstart your fitness journey. During these 30 days, you will have daily callisthenic workouts, walk 10,000 steps, follow our nutrition guidelines, and complete daily homework assignments. After completing the 30-day program, we offer an Omega program, which is an additional 60 days. This program builds upon the foundation established in the initial 30 days and provides further opportunities for growth and progress.

What is the cost of the program and are there any additional fees?
As of now, the cost of the program is already paid for with the purchase of the book for the initial 30-day challenge. There are no additional fees, and you will have access to all the resources and support throughout the program. To become a member beyond the wolf cubs there are membership options available, but let's get you passing the wolf cub phase first.

What kind of results can I expect to achieve by following the program?
While the program does include fitness and nutrition components, our main focus is on mental and emotional health and wellness. By following the program, you can expect to gain strength of mind and body, as well as improved self-confidence and overall well-being. While losing body fat and weight may be a positive side effect, it's important to remember that mental and emotional health are our top priorities. We believe that a healthy body and a healthy mind go hand in hand, and our program is designed to help you achieve both. So yes, we expect you can lose lots of fat, gain muscle and feel champion!

Can I still participate in the program if I have a pre-existing medical condition?
This is an important question, as we want to ensure that everyone can participate in the program safely. We encourage individuals with pre-existing medical conditions to consult with their healthcare provider before starting the program. It's important to understand any limitations or modifications that may need to be made to ensure your safety while participating in the program. Our program is designed to be customizable, so we can work with you and your healthcare provider to create a plan that is tailored to your needs and abilities. Your health and safety is our top priority, and we want to ensure that you can participate in the program in a safe and effective way.

Are there any age restrictions for the program?
Yes, there are age restrictions for the program. Participants must be at least 18 years old to join. This is because the program involves physical activity and may not be suitable for individuals under the age of 18. It is important to consult with a doctor or healthcare professional before starting any new exercise program.

How often should I weigh myself to track my progress?
It is recommended to not focus too much on the number on the scale as weight can fluctuate daily due to factors such as hydration and food intake. Instead, it may be more helpful to track progress by taking measurements, progress photos, and monitoring how your clothes fit. However, if weighing yourself is important to you, it is recommended to do so no more than once a week at the same time of day and under similar conditions.

Can I still drink alcohol or have cheat meals during the program?
No, during the initial 30-day program, you must not drink alcohol or have cheat meals. It is essential to stay committed and focused on your goals to achieve the best results. The program is designed to help you build healthy habits and make positive lifestyle changes, which requires discipline and consistency. However, if you decide to join the Omega pack level, we will slowly reintroduce social dynamics and drinking and making better choices for when to have a cheat meal, keeping in mind the fundamental question of "the one you feed," your light or your dark wolf.

What if I can't complete a workout due to physical limitations or lack of equipment?
If you have physical limitations or lack of equipment, there are modifications and alternative exercises that can be provided for you. It's important to communicate with your coach or trainer to let them know about any limitations or challenges you may be facing,

so they can provide you with appropriate modifications. Remember, the program is designed to be adaptable and accessible for all fitness levels and abilities. The key is to stay committed and consistent with the program, and to listen to your body to avoid injury.

Will I need to take supplements as part of the program?
We do not require participants to take any supplements as part of the program. However, we do provide guidance on how to make healthy food choices that can help you meet your nutritional needs. If you feel that you are lacking certain nutrients, we recommend consulting with a healthcare professional to determine if supplements may be necessary for you.

Can I still participate in other physical activities while doing this program?
Yes, you can still participate in other physical activities while doing this program. However, keep in mind that the program is designed to provide a comprehensive fitness and wellness experience, so it's important to listen to your body and ensure that you are not overexerting yourself or risking injury. Additionally, if you have any questions or concerns about how other physical activities may impact your progress in the program, it's recommended that you consult with a healthcare professional or certified personal trainer.

What happens if I get injured or miss a day due to a family emergency?
If you get injured or need to miss a day due to a family emergency, we recommend that you prioritize your health and safety first. It's important to listen to your body and not push yourself too hard if you're injured. If you do miss a workout or fall behind, don't worry. You can always make up for it the next day or adjust your schedule accordingly.

Remember, this program is designed to be flexible and adaptable to your needs. If you have any concerns or questions about modifications due to injury, please consult with your healthcare provider before continuing with the program.

What happens after the 30 day program is completed?
For those who want to continue their journey towards becoming the best version of themselves, we offer the Omega Pack, which is available for the price of a coffee each week. With the Omega Pack, you can continue with the program and receive ongoing support, guidance, and motivation. This pack includes an additional 60-day program that will help you build on the foundation you established during the initial 30-day program. It also provides access to exclusive content, such as live Q&A sessions with our trainers, recipe books, and much more. So, if you're serious about achieving your fitness and wellness goals and want to continue your journey with us, we invite you to join the Omega Pack.

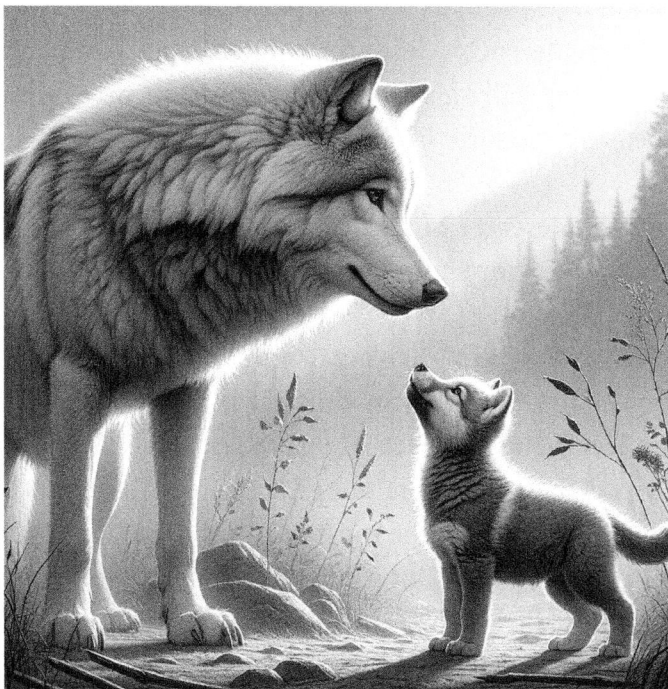

You in numbers

XXIII

As you prepare to journey through the Two Wolves program, the first step is to establish a clear and accurate starting point by documenting essential biomarkers. These metrics are pivotal in crafting a personalized path towards wellness, allowing you to track progress, adjust your strategy, and celebrate your successes with precision.

Key Biomarkers and How to Measure Them:
- **Weight**: Use a reliable scale on a flat surface. It's best to weigh yourself at the same time each day, preferably in the morning, to maintain consistency.
- **Body Fat Percentage**: For accuracy, consider using a body composition scale or a skinfold caliper. Follow the manufacturer's instructions carefully or seek assistance from a professional.
- **Waist Circumference:** Measure around the narrowest part of your waist, typically just above the belly button, using a flexible tape measure. Ensure the tape is snug but not compressing your skin.
- **Bicep Circumference:** Measure around the fullest part of your bicep with the arm relaxed at your side, using a flexible tape measure.
- **Thigh Circumference:** Measure around the fullest part of your thigh, close to the top, with your feet slightly apart.
- **Resting Heart Rate (RHR):** Measure your pulse first thing in the morning before getting out of bed. Count the number of beats in 60 seconds for the most accurate reading.
- **Blood Pressure:** Use a blood pressure monitor, following the instructions for use. It's best measured after resting for at least 5 minutes, seated in a calm environment.

- **Touch Toes (Flexibility):** Stand with your feet together and legs straight. Reach down towards your toes without bending your knees. Note the distance between your fingers and toes, or if you can touch or surpass your toes.
- **Mood Assessment:** Reflect on your overall mood and well-being. Consider using a scale from 1 to 10, with 1 being very poor mood and 10 being excellent. This subjective measure is crucial for acknowledging the mental and emotional starting point of your wellness journey.

While it may feel daunting to confront these metrics, remember that they are simply starting points. They provide a map from which your journey begins, not judgments of your current state. Honest accountability and self-compassion are the heart of the Two Wolves program, empowering you to own your journey and embrace growth.

Embracing Your Metrics with Purpose:
Recording these biomarkers does more than set benchmarks; it signifies a commitment to your health and an openness to change. Each metric, from physical measurements like waist circumference to subjective assessments like mood, offers insight into your holistic well-being.

As you document your starting points, approach the task with kindness and objectivity. These numbers are tools for self-improvement, not criticisms. They serve as the foundation upon which your progress is built, celebrated, and refined.

Throughout your transformation, revisit these biomarkers to marvel at how far you've come and to guide your path forward. In the Two Wolves program, every step taken, whether forward or backward, is part of the journey toward a healthier, happier you. This baseline is your launchpad to greatness, a testament to where you began and a beacon for where you're headed.

Biomarker Measurements

Date of Measurement: _____

_____ | **Weight**: Morning measurement before eating (lbs/kg).

_____ | **Body Fat %:** Use a scale or caliper (%).

_____ | **Waist Circumference**: Measure above the belly button (inches/cm).

_____ | **Bicep Circumference:** Measure the fullest part of the bicep (inches/cm).

_____ | **Thigh Circumference:** Measure the fullest part of the thigh (inches/cm).

_____ | **Resting Heart Rate:** Measure upon waking, count beats for 60 seconds (bpm).

_____ | **Blood Pressure:** Use a blood pressure monitor (mmHg).

_____ | **Touch Toes:** Can you touch your toes? Note the distance if not (Yes/No/Distance).

_____ | **Mood:** Rate on a scale of 1 being very poor mood, 10 being excellent (1-10 scale).

Instructions: Fill in the blanks with your initial measurements to establish a baseline for your progress. This structured approach allows you to monitor improvements and adapt your journey as needed, fostering a path toward holistic wellness.

Wolf Tracker I

XXIV

Welcome to the cornerstone of your transformation journey—the Wolf Tracker: Fitness Assessment. This pivotal evaluation, woven into our 30-day program, serves as both a starting point and a continual gauge of your growth. By engaging in a series of four exercises, we'll capture a snapshot of your current fitness level, setting the stage for measurable progress and providing the impetus for you to exceed your own expectations.

Our assessment kicks off with the pushup challenge, inviting you to complete as many pushups as you can within a span of one minute. Following a brief five-minute interlude to recover, we'll shift our focus to the squat challenge, again testing your strength and endurance over another minute. The third trial, the jumping jack challenge, continues to assess your cardiovascular fitness and agility in a one-minute burst. Lastly, after a final five-minute pause for recovery, we dive into the elbow plank challenge, a true test of your core strength and endurance as you hold the plank position for as long as possible.

Your achievements in each exercise will be meticulously documented on the accompanying worksheet, which you're encouraged to revisit and update every seven days. Witnessing your own evolution over the course of the program—not just from week to week but cumulatively over the full 30 days—is both inspiring and affirming.

It's crucial to remember that the essence of this journey lies not in the numbers themselves but in the progress they represent. Each step forward, no matter the size, marks a triumph in the quest to unveil the best version of yourself.

No matter your starting point—be it a single pushup or a marathon of them—this moment, day zero, is the beginning of your metamorphosis. By day 30, the transformation in your physical capabilities will be palpable, a testament to your dedication and hard work.

Embrace this process with an open heart and steadfast commitment. Trust in the journey ahead, for within you stirs the spirit of the wolf, ready to emerge stronger, more resilient, and triumphant. Awoo!

1. Push Ups:
- **How to Perform:** Start in a high plank position with your hands firmly on the ground, directly under your shoulders. Keeping your body in a straight line, lower yourself until your chest nearly touches the floor. Push back up to the starting position.
- **Scoring Area:**
  - **Day 1 Score:** _____ push-ups in one minute
  - **Notes:** _____

2. Squats:
- **How to Perform:** Stand with your feet shoulder-width apart, toes slightly pointed out. Bend your knees and push your hips back as if sitting in a chair, keeping your chest up and knees over your toes. Push through your heels to return to standing.
- **Scoring Area:**
  - **Day 1 Score:** _____ squats in one minute
  - **Notes:** _____

3. Jumping Jacks:

- **How to Perform:** Stand upright with your legs together, arms at your sides. Jump up, spreading your legs shoulder-width apart while simultaneously raising your arms above your head. Jump back to the starting position.
- **Scoring Area:**
  - **Day 1 Score:** _____ jumping jacks in one minute
  - **Notes:** _____

4. Plank:

- **How to Perform:** Begin in the forearm plank position with your elbows on the ground directly under your shoulders, legs extended behind you. Engage your core, ensuring your body forms a straight line from head to heels. Hold this position.
- **Scoring Area:**
  - **Day 1 Score:** _____ time held in plank
  - **Notes:** _____

Instructions for Use: As you tackle each exercise, record your scores diligently, noting the number of repetitions or the duration you've managed to achieve. Revisit and update your scores weekly to monitor your progress, reflecting on any adjustments or improvements needed. Remember, this journey is uniquely yours— every effort made, every boundary pushed, brings you one step closer to the strength and resilience emblematic of the wolf spirit within.

Let the Wolf Tracker 1 be both your starting line and your guidepost, marking your progress as you journey through the 30-day challenge. Trust in your growth, celebrate your achievements, and push forward with the heart of a wolf. Awoo!

  o

A Wolf Is Born

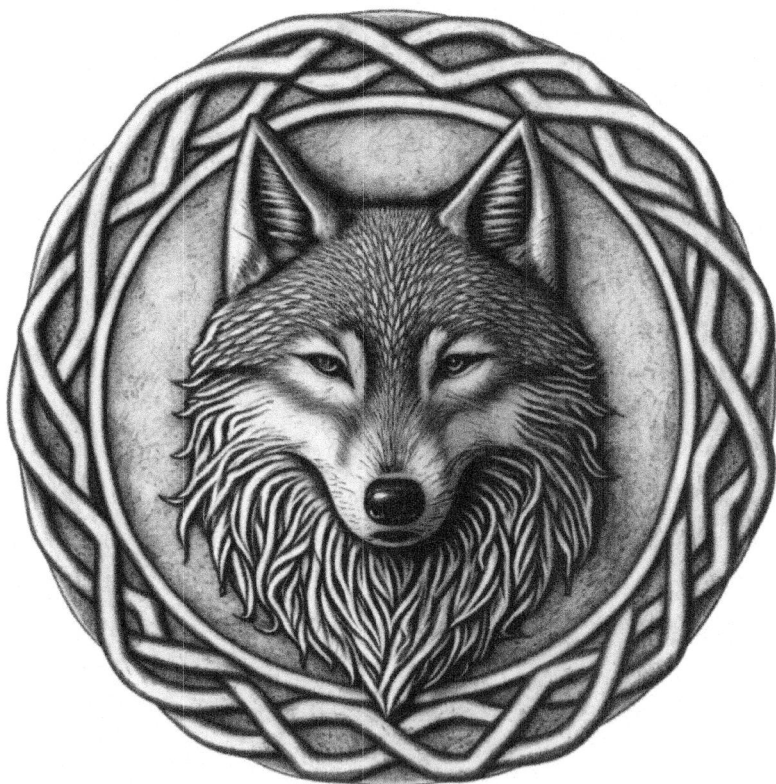

Let's Begin...

How to use this workbook

This book is designed not just as a guide but as a companion through the 30-day challenge, offering daily "packwork" - insights, encouragement, and thought-provoking prompts to guide your path.

You might notice some themes or messages appearing more than once throughout this book. This is intentional. Repetition is not just a method of teaching; it is a way of embedding values and understanding deep within us. Each repeated lesson is a layer, adding depth to your foundation, ensuring that the principles of resilience, strength, and wisdom are not merely understood but lived and breathed.

At the end of each day's passage, you will find three questions. These are designed to provoke thought, reflection, and deeper understanding. Writing down your thoughts helps to access deeper realms of consciousness, making the lessons not just read but experienced and internalized.

Beyond these questions, the book offers space for you to journal your journey. This is your private sanctuary to express your thoughts on progress, worries, anxieties, and breakthroughs. Journaling is a powerful tool for self-discovery, allowing you to see your growth over time and confront the challenges with honesty and courage.

You are encouraged, though never obligated, to share your journaling with the pack. The community created around this challenge is a source of accountability and encouragement. Sharing your journey can not only help you but also inspire others in the pack. Your story could be the key that unlocks someone else's potential.

This book is your White Wolf, a guiding light through each day of the challenge. It is here to provide support, wisdom, and encouragement as you navigate the path ahead. To maximize the results of these 30 days, engage with each element of the book fully. Use it to reflect, to learn, and to grow. The journey ahead is yours, and every page turned is another step towards becoming the best version of yourself.

Embrace the journey with an open heart and a willing spirit. The next 30 days have the power to change your life. Let this book be your guide, your mentor, and your friend as you embark on this journey. Welcome to the pack, and remember, this is only the beginning. The path to becoming your best self is a lifelong journey, and it starts right now.

Phase I

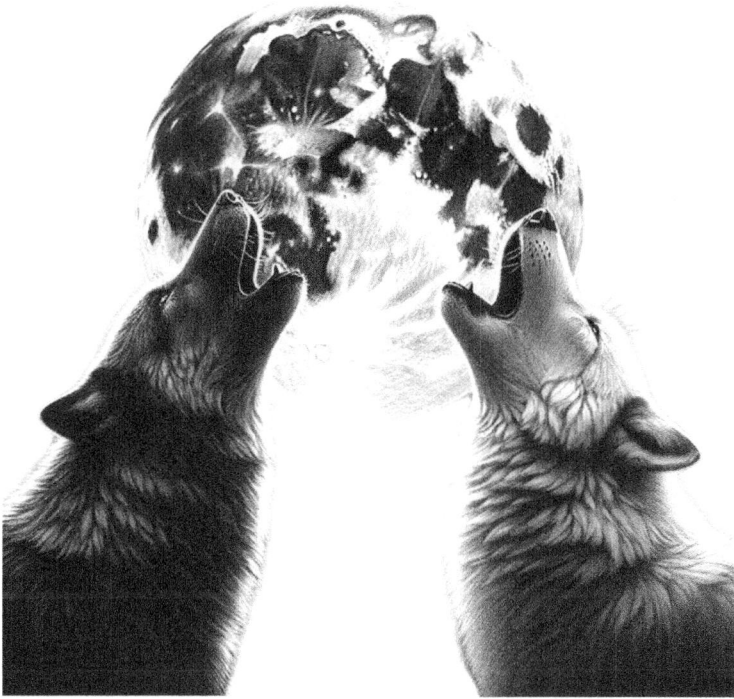

Foundations

Day 1 Chapter 1
A Wolf is Born

"Throw me to the wolves and I will return leading the pack."
- *Unknown*

As dusk falls and the celestial dance of the night sky unfolds, the resonant howl of a newborn wolf pierces the tranquil silence, heralding its entry into the world. This primal anthem speaks of resilience, of a relentless spirit woven into the very fabric of the wilderness. The wolf, a paragon of tenacity, loyalty, and formidable strength, traverses the landscape with grace, hunts with unmatched precision, and thrives through unity with its pack. It embodies the essence of survival, adaptation, and the sheer will to prevail against all odds. This symbol of endurance and the collective power of the pack now also represents you.

The Two Wolves program is meticulously crafted to awaken your intrinsic capabilities, to guide you through life's adversities, and to foster a transformation that sees you emerge with newfound wisdom, fortitude, and an indomitable spirit. Rooted in the ancient parable of the two wolves battling within us—one representing fear and doubt, the other courage and hope—our journey hinges on which wolf we choose to nurture.

Embarking on this journey through the Four Phases of the Two Wolves program, you will cultivate the virtues of the noble wolf within—courage, self-assurance, and optimism. This path is designed not only to inspire you to seize the reins of your destiny, to chase after your dreams with fervor, and to surmount the hurdles in your path but is also anchored in scientific rigor and the timeless wisdom of our ancestors.

As you stand at the threshold of this transformative adventure, know that you are joining a lineage of individuals who, like you, sought to harness their latent potential. These individuals, guided by the principles of this program, have rekindled their purpose, fortified their self-belief, and deepened their connection to their primal essence.

Welcome to the pack. Together, we will serenade the moon, navigate the challenges that lie ahead, champion our triumphs, tame the cacophony of self-doubt, and cultivate an oasis of self-compassion. In unison, we will refine our ability to stride with purpose, to hunt our aspirations with precision, and to embody the elegance and grace of the wolf.

In the face of skepticism or the temptation to dismiss this journey as mere fantasy, we invite you to open your heart to the transformative power of this experience. Venturing into the unknown, embracing the discomfort of growth, is the crucible in which true change is forged. This program, a convergence of evidence-based methodologies and spiritual wisdom, has catalyzed the metamorphosis of many before you.

Are you prepared to heed the primal call to adventure, to unlock the wolf within? The wild beckons, Cub. Let us embark on this odyssey together. Awoo!

"Change is the end result of all true learning." - Leo Buscaglia.

Armed with this knowledge, are you ready to embark on a journey of profound learning and transformation?

Daily Checklist (tick off)

☐ Meditation
☐ 10,000 Steps & Proof
☐ Wolf Workout
☐ Water Intake
☐ 8-Hour Eating Window
☐ Daily Learning (*Homework*)
☐ Supplements (*Optional*)
☐ 7+ Hours of Sleep
☐ Daily Progress Photo
☐ Alcohol & Sugar-Free

1. What qualities, habits, and beliefs define who you are today?

_____

_____

_____

_____

_____

2. Who do you aspire to become by the end of this challenge?

_____

_____

_____

_____

_____

3. What specific steps will you take to transform from your current self to your ideal self?

_____

_____

_____

_____

Journal the journey

Journal your thoughts on how you feel today and what steps you'll take to succeed tomorrow.

_____
_____
_____
_____
_____
_____
_____
_____
_____
_____
_____
_____
_____
_____
_____
_____
_____
_____
_____
_____
_____
_____
_____
_____
_____
_____
_____
_____
_____
_____
_____
_____
_____

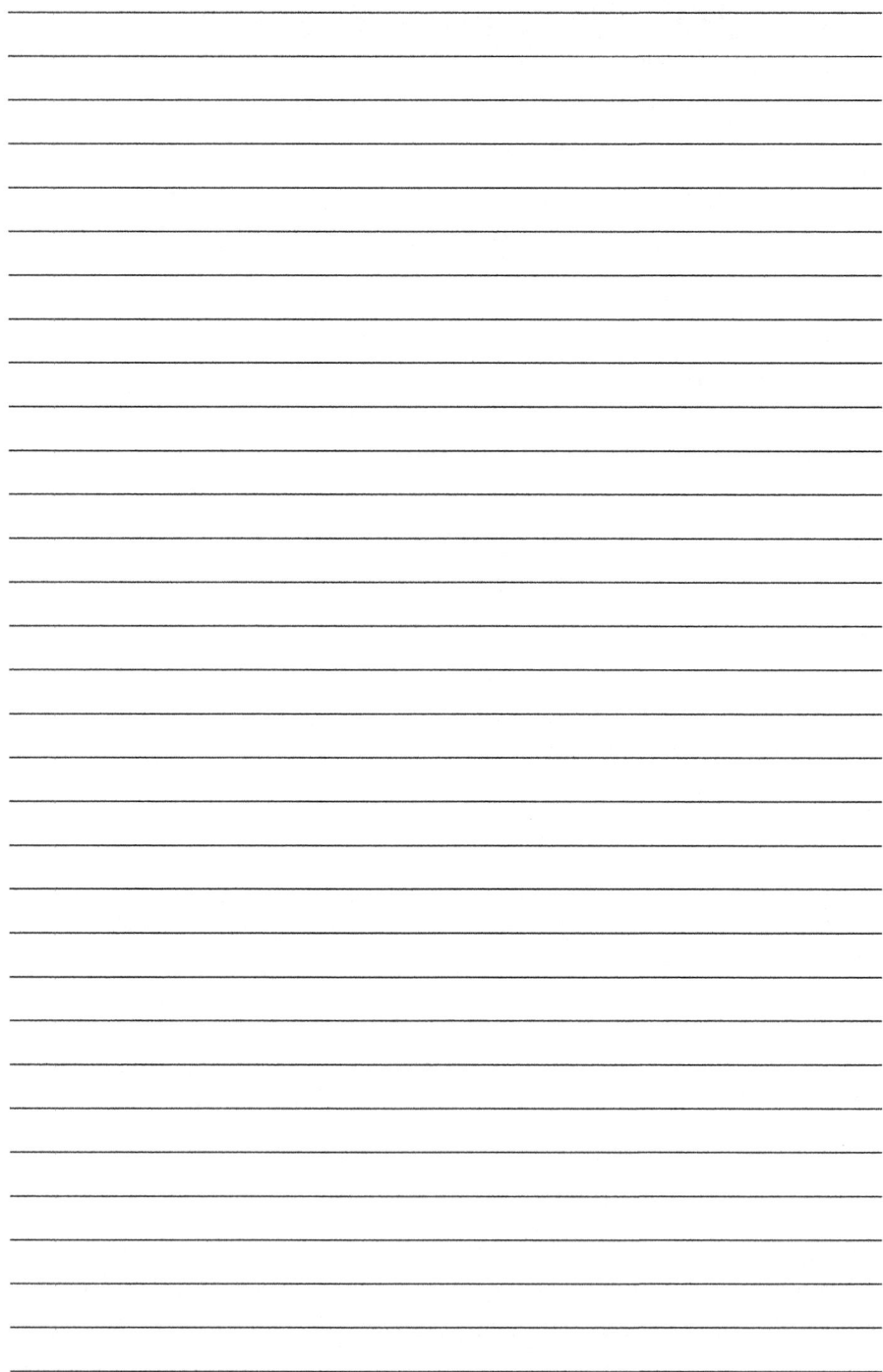

Day 2 Chapter 2
The Power of Mindset

"The mind is everything. What you think, you become."
- Buddha

In the evolving narrative of human potential, the power of mindset emerges as the pivotal force shaping our lives. It's a concept championed by modern-day philosophers, scientists, and wellness experts, who collectively underscore the profound impact our mental framework has on our health, achievements, and overall quality of life. Alongside Aubrey Marcus, Dr. Andrew Huberman, and Wim Hof, figures like Brené Brown offer compelling insights into the transformative potential of embracing vulnerability and resilience.

Brené Brown: A research professor who has spent her career studying courage, vulnerability, shame, and empathy, Brown advocates for the strength found in embracing our vulnerabilities. *"Vulnerability is not winning or losing; it's having the courage to show up and be seen when we have no control over the outcome,"* she asserts. This idea resonates deeply with the journey of feeding the right wolf, emphasizing that true growth comes from confronting our fears and stepping into the arena, regardless of the outcome.

Aubrey Marcus: A proponent of holistic well-being, Marcus emphasizes the synergy between mind, body, and spirit. *"We are each born with a unique potential that argues against the confines of our limiting beliefs,"* Marcus asserts. His approach champions the establishment of daily rituals that foster a state of readiness and resilience, such as setting intentions that act as a compass for our thoughts and actions.

Dr. Andrew Huberman: Huberman's research into neuroplasticity and the brain's adaptability offers a beacon of hope for those looking to transform their mindset. *"Your brain is constantly remodeling itself based on your experiences... You have the power to shape those experiences,"* he states. Huberman advocates for specific practices like focused breathing and light exposure to manipulate our physiological states, thereby inducing mental clarity and reducing stress.

Wim Hof: Known for his almost superhuman ability to withstand extreme cold, Hof has revolutionized our understanding of the mind-body connection. *"The cold is merciless but righteous,"* Hof proclaims, teaching that through the deliberate application of cold exposure, controlled breathing, and mental focus, we can unlock previously untapped reserves of strength and endurance.

The synthesis of these perspectives paints a compelling picture of mindset as the foundation upon which we can build a life of fulfillment and purpose. The dialogue between ancient wisdom and modern science offers actionable strategies for cultivating a mindset poised for growth, resilience, and transformation.

Expanding Your Mental Horizons: Key Practices
- **Adopt a Growth Mindset:** Inspired by the work of Carol Dweck, embrace challenges as opportunities for growth. View failures not as insurmountable obstacles but as valuable lessons that inform your journey.
- **Mindful Meditation:** Incorporate meditation practices into your daily routine to enhance self-awareness and reduce stress. Visualization techniques, such as the Wolf Meditation, can reinforce your connection to your inner strength and resilience.
- **Cultivate Gratitude:** Echoing the practices recommended by thought leaders across disciplines, maintain a gratitude journal. Documenting moments of gratitude shifts your focus from scarcity to abundance, fostering a more positive outlook on life.

- **Harness the Power of Breath:** Drawing from Huberman and Hof, utilize breathing exercises to regulate your nervous system. This simple yet profound practice can dramatically improve your emotional and physical well-being.
- **Embrace Physical Challenges:** Whether it's through cold exposure or engaging in regular physical activity, challenge your body to reinforce the mind-body connection. This physical resilience mirrors the mental strength you are developing.
- **Foster Positive Relationships:** Surround yourself with a supportive community that uplifts and motivates you. The energy and attitudes of those around us can significantly influence our mindset and vice versa.
- **Continuous Learning:** Commit to lifelong learning and curiosity. Engage with new ideas, skills, and experiences to keep your mind sharp and adaptable.

By weaving these practices into the tapestry of our daily lives, we unlock the door to a realm of possibilities previously confined by the limitations of a fixed mindset. The journey through the Two Wolves program is just the beginning; the true power of mindset unfolds as we apply these principles beyond the program, into every facet of our existence.

Remember, *"The mind is like a parachute. It doesn't work if it is not open."* - Frank Zappa.

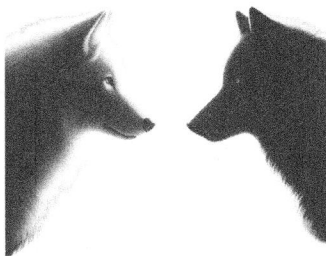

Daily Checklist (tick off)

☐ Meditation

☐ 10,000 Steps & Proof

☐ Wolf Workout

☐ Water Intake

☐ 8-Hour Eating Window

☐ Daily Learning (*Homework*)

☐ Supplements (*Optional*)

☐ 7+ Hours of Sleep

☐ Daily Progress Photo

☐ Alcohol & Sugar-Free

1. What change do you hope to see in yourself by adopting a growth mindset?

_____

_____

_____

_____

_____

2. How does the idea of vulnerability as a strength resonate with your personal journey?

_____

_____

_____

_____

_____

3. Which daily habit will you start today to positively shift your mindset?

_____

_____

_____

_____

date ___ / ___ / ___

Journal the journey

Journal your thoughts on how you feel today and what steps you'll take to succeed tomorrow.

_____
_____
_____
_____
_____
_____
_____
_____
_____
_____
_____
_____
_____
_____
_____
_____
_____
_____
_____
_____
_____
_____
_____
_____
_____
_____
_____
_____
_____
_____
_____
_____
_____
_____
_____
_____

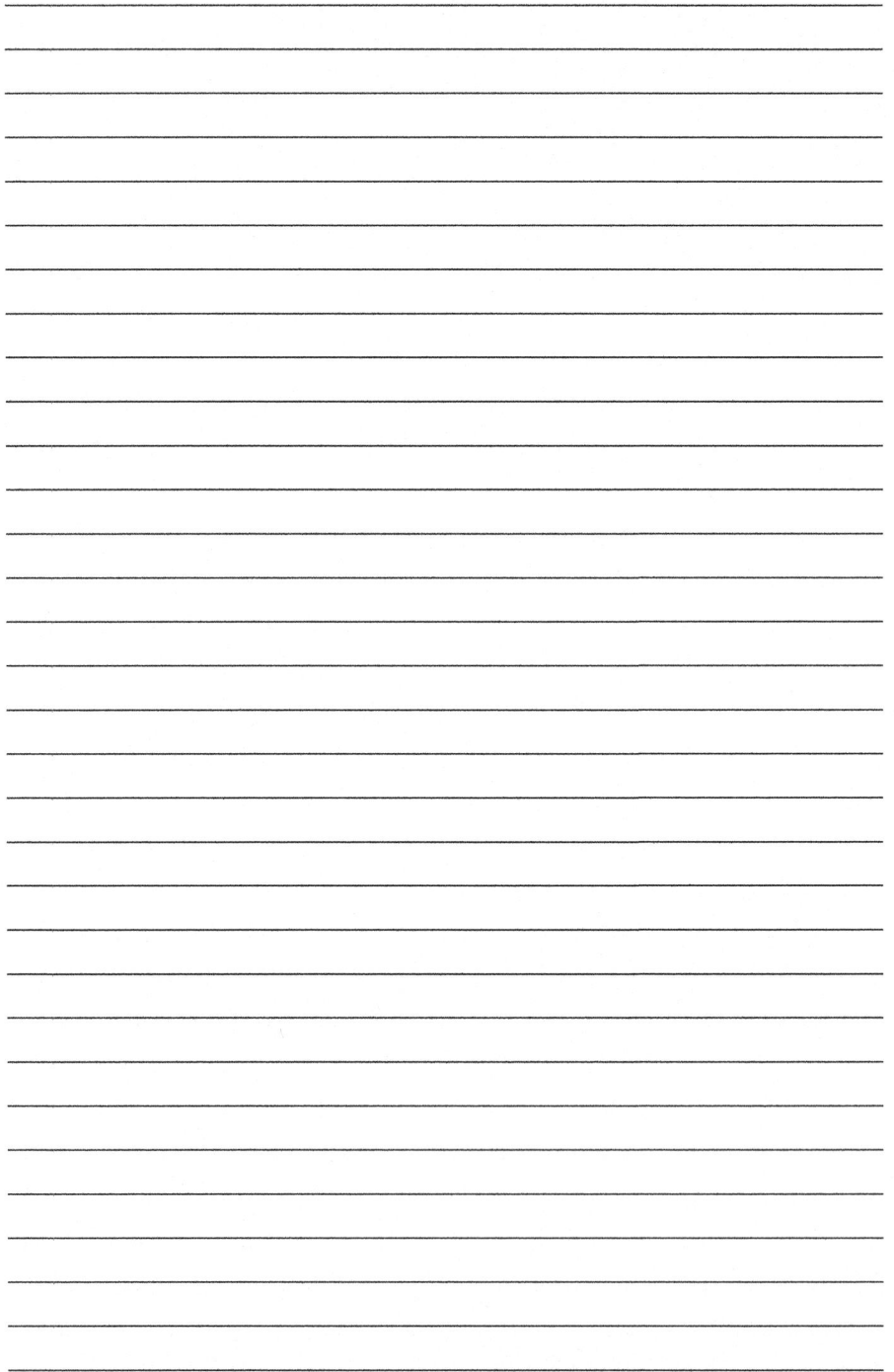

Day 3 Chapter 3
Identifying & Overcoming Self Doubt

"Believe you can and you're halfway there."
- Theodore Roosevelt

Embarking on the journey to dismantle self-doubt is akin to navigating through a dense, uncharted forest. It's a terrain fraught with the whispers of past failures, the shadows of inadequacy, and the echoes of missed opportunities. Yet, within this forest lies the path to our true potential, waiting to be uncovered and traversed. Self-doubt, by its very nature, is an insidious force; it seeps into the crevices of our psyche, often masquerading as a protective voice, a guardian against the perils of risk and vulnerability. However, this guise is misleading, for it is not protection but a prison, crafted from the chains of our fears and insecurities.

To truly understand and conquer self-doubt, we must first acknowledge its complexity. It is not merely a surface-level adversary, easily vanquished with a few words of encouragement or a single act of defiance. Rather, it is a deeply ingrained pattern of thought, nurtured by years of conditioning and experiences that have taught us to question our worth, our abilities, and our right to aspire. Modern psychological research sheds light on this phenomenon, illustrating how self-doubt can significantly impact our decision-making processes, creativity, and willingness to engage in new and challenging experiences. Cognitive Behavioral Therapy (CBT) and other therapeutic approaches have underscored the power of identifying and challenging these negative thought patterns, offering evidence-based strategies for individuals seeking to reclaim their minds from the grip of doubt.

The journey of overcoming self-doubt is, therefore, both a battle and a rebirth. It requires a deep dive into the self, a willingness to confront and understand the origins of our doubts, and an unwavering commitment to forging a new narrative. This process is akin to the ancient practice of alchemy, where base metals were believed to be transformed into gold. Here, the base metal is our self-doubt, and the gold is the untapped potential that lies within each of us, waiting to be discovered and realized.

In this chapter, we will explore the multifaceted nature of self-doubt, drawing on the wisdom of ancient philosophers, the insights of modern-day thought leaders, and the findings of contemporary scientific research. Together, these perspectives will guide us on a journey of transformation—a journey from doubt to certainty, from fear to courage, and from stagnation to growth.

The labyrinth of self-doubt is a formidable barrier to personal evolution, ensnaring us in its web of insecurity and hesitation. Yet, history and modern science alike offer us keys to liberation, showing us how to dismantle these barriers with the precision of a skilled architect.

Understanding Self-Doubt: Self-doubt often disguises itself as a voice of reason, masquerading as prudent caution. Yet, beneath this guise lies a torrent of limiting beliefs that stifle our potential. Identifying self-doubt is the inaugural step in our journey towards emancipation. Neuroscience illuminates this path, revealing how our brain patterns can be rewired through consistent, positive mental practices. Dr. Carol Dweck's pioneering work on the growth mindset underscores this, illustrating how embracing challenges, effort, and mistakes as avenues for learning can transform our approach to personal and professional obstacles.

The Pillar of Self-Compassion: Kristin Neff, a leading researcher on self-compassion, articulates the transformative power of treating oneself with kindness during moments of failure. She notes, *"Self-compassion is not self-pity, but rather a self-kindness that recognizes the universality of our human experience."* Embracing our flaws and setbacks with empathy and understanding fosters a resilient growth mindset, propelling us beyond the confines of self-doubt.

Nurturing a Supportive Ecosystem: The ancient proverb, *"You are the average of the five people you spend the most time with,"* attributed to Jim Rohn, emphasizes the influence of our social circles on our mindset. Cultivating relationships with individuals who embody the traits we aspire to can significantly diminish self-doubt, replacing it with contagious confidence. These relationships act as mirrors, reflecting back our potential and worth, thus fortifying our resolve against the whisperings of self-doubt.

Embracing Risk and Reframing Failure: The narrative of failure in our society is undergoing a radical transformation, spearheaded by thought leaders like Brené Brown, who champions vulnerability and courage. *"There is no innovation and creativity without failure. Period,"* Brown asserts. This perspective invites us to reconceptualize failure not as a verdict on our worth but as vital feedback in our journey of growth and discovery.

The Choice of Perspective: At the crux of overcoming self-doubt lies the decision of which wolf we choose to feed within us—despair or hope, stagnation or growth. This decision shapes our reality, molding our experiences and outcomes. Marcus Aurelius, the Stoic philosopher, once said, *"Our life is what our thoughts make it."* Embracing this wisdom, we recognize the power of mindset as the architect of our destiny.

Feeding the right wolf requires a daily commitment to positive self-talk, challenging our limitations, and stepping into the unknown with the courage of a warrior. It involves leaning into discomfort, knowing that the alchemy of growth occurs in the crucible of challenge.

As we navigate the terrain of self-doubt, let us arm ourselves with the lessons of those who have walked this path before us, drawing from the wells of ancient wisdom and modern science. The journey is fraught with trials, but each step forward is a victory in the quest for self-realization and fulfillment.

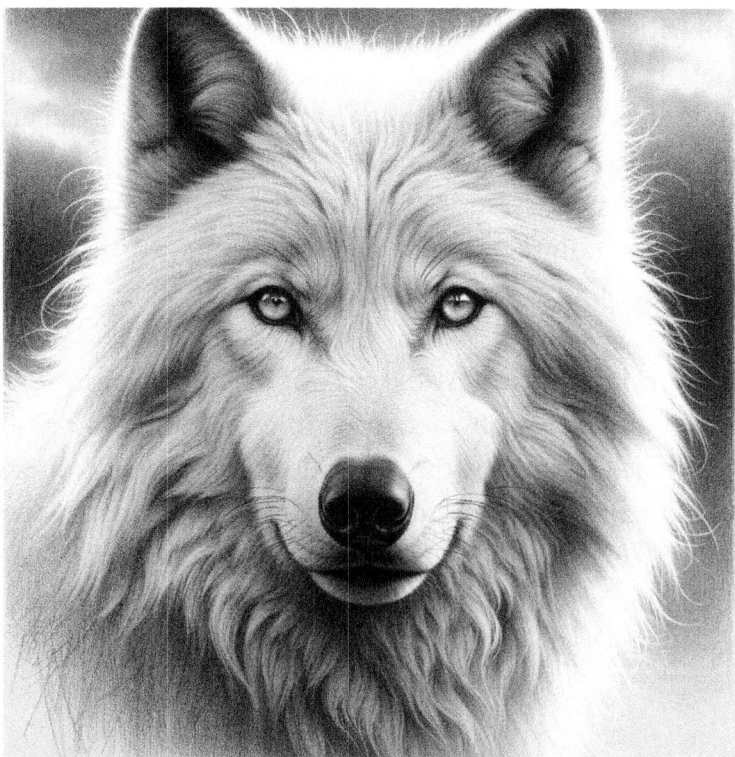

Daily Checklist (tick off)

☐ Meditation
☐ 10,000 Steps & Proof
☐ Wolf Workout
☐ Water Intake
☐ 8-Hour Eating Window
☐ Daily Learning (*Homework*)
☐ Supplements (*Optional*)
☐ 7+ Hours of Sleep
☐ Daily Progress Photo
☐ Alcohol & Sugar-Free

1. What specific thought patterns of self-doubt do you recognize in yourself, and how can you challenge them starting today?

_____

_____

_____

_____

_____

2. Can you identify one action you've hesitated to take due to self-doubt? How can you approach it differently with a growth mindset?

_____

_____

_____

_____

_____

3. Reflecting on your support system, how can you actively seek or strengthen relationships that encourage your confidence and growth?

_____

_____

_____

Journal the journey

Journal your thoughts on how you feel today and what steps you'll take to succeed tomorrow.

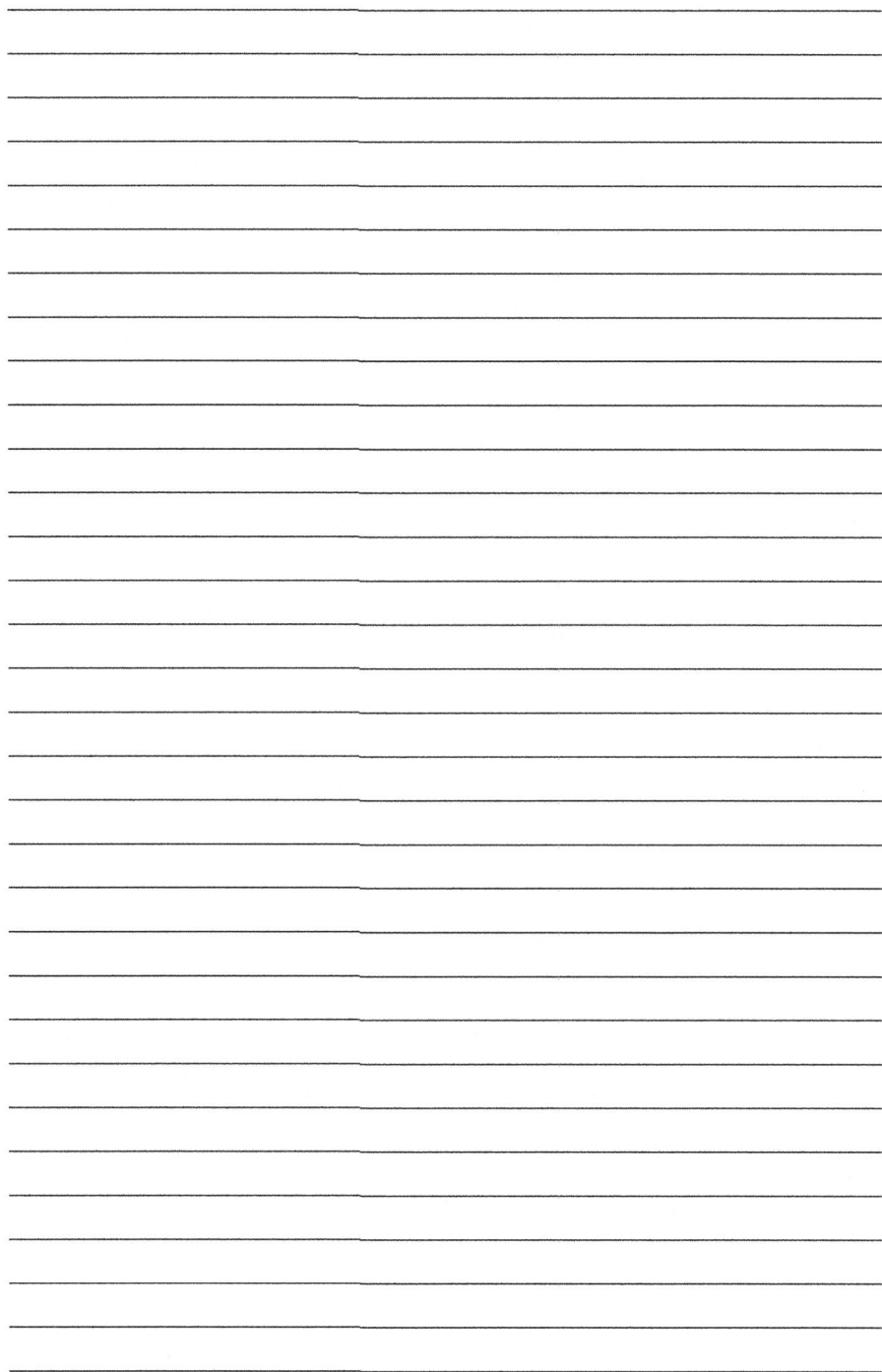

Day 4 Chapter 4
The Role of Nutrition

"Let food be thy medicine and medicine be thy food."
- Hippocrates

In the grand odyssey of achieving optimal health and vitality, nutrition stands as the bedrock upon which all else is built. It is not merely about the sustenance required for survival but a sophisticated interplay between what we consume and how it fuels the myriad functions of our bodies. This chapter delves into the profound impact of nutrition on physical fitness, echoing the wisdom of ancient philosophers and corroborating with the findings of modern science to guide you on a path of informed dietary choices.

A Dialogue Across Millennia: Ancient Wisdom Meets Modern Science: The ancient Greeks, with Hippocrates at the helm, posited nutrition as the cornerstone of health, a concept that resonates through centuries into our current understanding of wellness. The Ayurvedic tradition, with its intricate classification of food types, also emphasizes the importance of dietary balance in maintaining physical and spiritual equilibrium. In parallel, contemporary research substantiates these ancient beliefs, demonstrating the undeniable link between nutrition and health outcomes. Journals such as The American Journal of Clinical Nutrition have published numerous studies highlighting how a balanced diet influences everything from cognitive function to physical resilience, underscoring nutrition's pivotal role in wellness.

Macronutrients: The Fuel for Life's Endeavors: The body's need for macronutrients—carbohydrates, proteins, and fats—is a testament to their essential role in our health.

Carbohydrates, the primary source of energy, are crucial for fueling both mental and physical activities, supporting everything from rigorous exercise to basic cognitive functions. Proteins, the building blocks of muscle, not only facilitate recovery and growth but also play a role in hormonal and enzyme functions critical to health. Fats, often misunderstood, are vital for cellular integrity, hormone production, and nutrient absorption. The International Society of Sports Nutrition provides a nuanced view of how these macronutrients support athletic performance and recovery, advocating for a balanced intake tailored to individual needs.

Hydration: The Wellspring of Vitality: The essence of life, water, is fundamental to our very existence. Hydration goes beyond quenching thirst; it is vital for maintaining body temperature, ensuring the transportation of nutrients, and facilitating cellular processes. The European Journal of Clinical Nutrition emphasizes the critical nature of hydration in physical performance, highlighting how even slight dehydration can impair strength, endurance, and mental acuity. This underscores the necessity of regular fluid intake, particularly for those engaged in physical activities.

Micronutrients: The Subtle Architects of Health: Micronutrients, though required in minute amounts, wield immense influence over our health. They catalyze biochemical reactions, support immune function, and contribute to bone density, among countless other roles. Iron, for instance, is indispensable for oxygen transport, while vitamin D plays a crucial role in calcium absorption and immune function. The diversity of micronutrients and their myriad functions underscores the importance of a varied diet, rich in fruits, vegetables, lean proteins, and healthy fats, to ensure adequate intake.

Embracing a Mindful Relationship with Food: Nutrition transcends the physical aspects of food intake, venturing into the psychological realm of our relationship with food. Mindful eating encourages an intentional and appreciative approach to meals, fostering a deep connection with the act of nourishing our bodies. This perspective transforms eating from a mundane task into a ritual of self-care, promoting a balanced and healthy relationship with food.

The Symphony of Balanced Nutrition: Achieving nutritional balance is akin to orchestrating a symphony, where each nutrient plays its part in harmony with others. Consistency in consuming a variety of whole foods ensures a steady supply of essential nutrients, supporting bodily functions and contributing to overall well-being. Regular, balanced meals fuel our daily activities, support long-term health, and enable us to engage with life fully.

In embracing the comprehensive view of nutrition outlined in this chapter, you embark on a journey not just toward physical health, but toward a profound transformation that touches every aspect of your being. It's a journey of discovery, where food becomes more than mere fuel—it becomes a source of joy, a medium of healing, and a path to realizing the fullest expression of ourselves.

"To eat is a necessity, but to eat intelligently is an art."
- François de La Rochefoucauld

Daily Checklist (tick off)
- ☐ Meditation
- ☐ 10,000 Steps & Proof
- ☐ Wolf Workout
- ☐ Water Intake
- ☐ 8-Hour Eating Window
- ☐ Daily Learning (*Homework*)
- ☐ Supplements (*Optional*)
- ☐ 7+ Hours of Sleep
- ☐ Daily Progress Photo
- ☐ Alcohol & Sugar-Free

How can integrating the practice of mindful eating transform your relationship with food and, subsequently, your overall well-being?

_____

_____

_____

_____

_____

What specific change will you make to your nutrition tomorrow to move closer to your wellness goals?

_____

_____

_____

_____

_____

What item can you remove from your pantry today and replace with a healthier alternative to support your nutritional goals?

_____

_____

_____

_____

Journal the journey

Journal your thoughts on how you feel today and what steps you'll take to succeed tomorrow.

_____

_____

_____

_____

_____

_____

_____

_____

_____

_____

_____

_____

_____

_____

_____

_____

_____

_____

_____

_____

_____

_____

_____

_____

_____

_____

_____

_____

_____

_____

_____

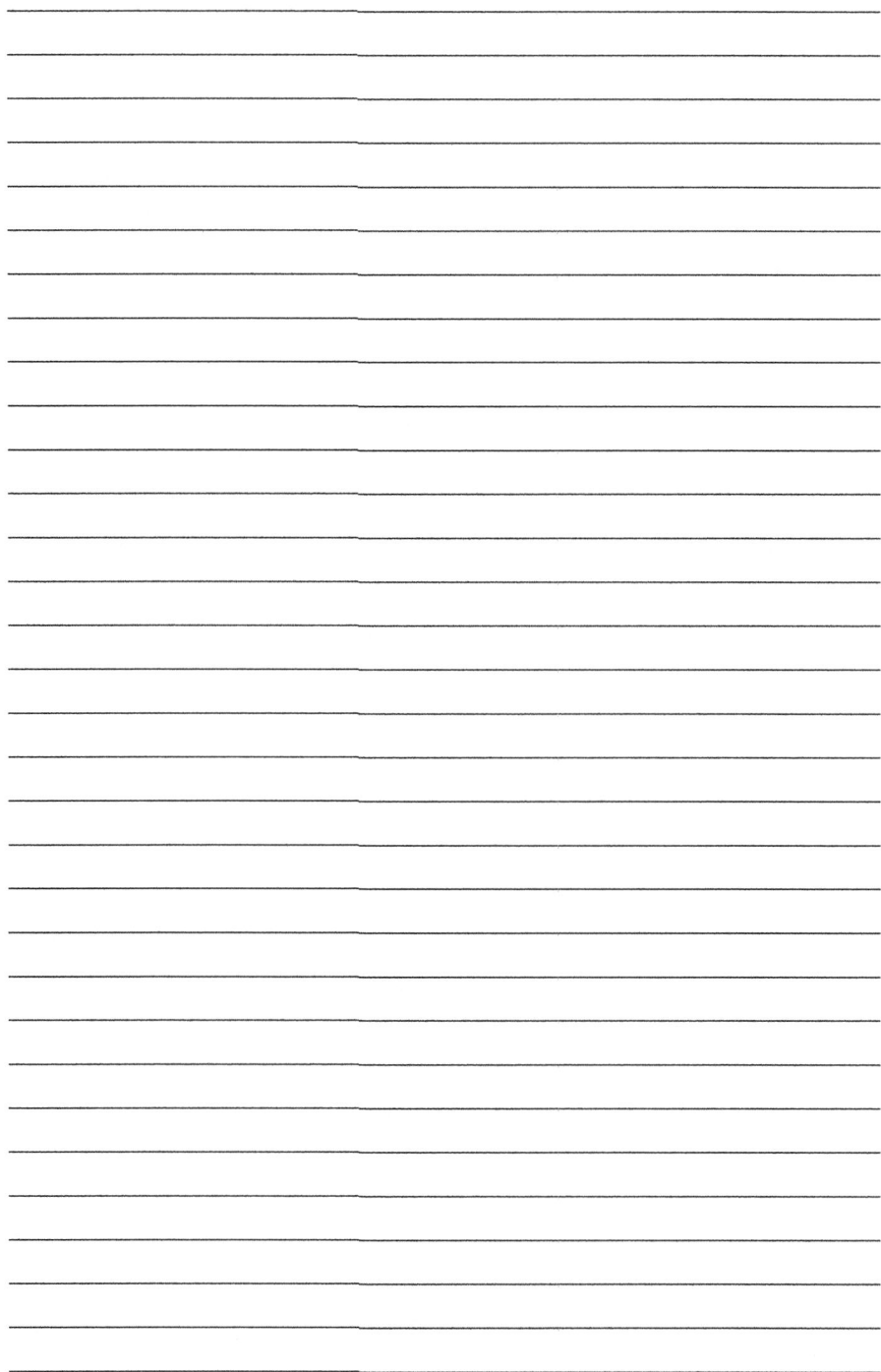

Day 5 Chapter 5
Building an effective routine

"The secret of your future is hidden in your daily routine."
- Mike Murdock

The architecture of our days is constructed from the routines and habits we cultivate. These routines not only define our daily actions but also sculpt our long-term health, happiness, and achievement. Mastering the art of establishing a life-enhancing routine can unlock extraordinary potential, guiding you towards the zenith of your capabilities.

The challenge many face in forging a productive routine stems from a lack of understanding of habit's transformative power. Habits, the subtle threads woven through the fabric of our daily existence, are forged through the fires of repetition. Each action, repeated, becomes a stitch in the tapestry of our subconscious, automating our behaviors and liberating mental resources for higher pursuits.
Yet, the spectrum of habits spans from the detrimental to the divine. Discerning which habits uplift and which ones hinder is crucial in crafting an effective routine. An empowering routine melds habits that nourish your body, enrich your mind, and soothe your soul, setting a foundation for holistic well-being.

The genesis of a life-enhancing routine begins with introspection and intention. Dismantling barriers requires a candid evaluation of your current habits—identifying those that serve as anchors and those that act as wings.

This reflective process is a journey into the heart of your desires and fears, demanding courage and commitment. Daily reflections, such as noting a "win" in your packwork, are vital in maintaining this introspective practice.

Planning is the next step in this journey of transformation. A robust routine is not a random assortment of tasks but a carefully curated collection of actions aligned with your deepest aspirations. This plan should harmonize with your physical, mental, and emotional rhythms, offering a balanced diet of activities that foster growth in every aspect of your being.

The linchpin of routine mastery is unwavering consistency. The initial phase of adopting a new routine might be strewn with challenges and discomfort, yet persistence paves the path to habituation. Over time, what once required conscious effort becomes second nature, a part of your essence.

An effective routine is a catalyst for positive momentum, igniting a chain reaction of beneficial choices throughout your day. It equips you with resilience against life's adversities, enhances your ability to manage stress, and unlocks unparalleled productivity. Starting your day with a sequence of actions that invigorate and prepare you for the challenges ahead can have a ripple effect, influencing every decision thereafter.

It's imperative to recognize that there is no universal blueprint for an effective routine. Your routine should be a reflection of your unique journey, adaptable to life's inevitable ebbs and flows. It is a living entity, evolving as you evolve, always in service of your highest good.

In the alchemy of self-transformation, establishing a life-enhancing routine is among the most potent tools at your disposal. By weaving positive habits into the fabric of your daily life, you initiate a process of continuous improvement. Embrace the power of habit, commit to your chosen routine, and bear witness to the unfolding of your potential. Remember, the magic is not in the routine itself, but in your dedication to it.

Tips to building your effective routine:

- **Define Clear Objectives:** Begin by setting specific, achievable goals. Knowing what you aim to achieve with your routine—be it better health, mental clarity, or productivity—provides direction and purpose.
- **Embrace Holistic Wellness:** A balanced routine addresses your physical, mental, and emotional needs. Incorporate exercise, mindfulness practices, intellectual challenges, and activities that bring joy, sharing your experiences with the wolf pack for encouragement and advice.
- **Start Small for Big Success:** Initiate your routine with small, manageable changes. Sharing these steps with the Two Wolves community can offer accountability and celebrate your progress, no matter how minor it may seem.
- **Strategically Schedule:** Plan your routine as diligently as any important appointment, and share your schedule with the wolf pack for additional accountability. This can help in maintaining consistency and receiving support when adjusting to new habits.
- **Align with Your Energy:** Craft your routine around your natural energy fluctuations. Share tips with the wolf pack on how to identify and utilize peak energy times for different activities.

- **Incorporate Recovery:** Ensure your routine includes sufficient sleep and relaxation to foster recovery. The wolf pack can be a great resource for sharing relaxation techniques and sleep hygiene tips.
- **Nutrition and Hydration:** Integrate mindful eating and adequate hydration into your daily routine, utilizing the wolf pack to exchange healthy recipes and hydration reminders to keep each other on track.
- **Allow for Flexibility:** Life's unpredictability means your routine should adapt as necessary. Use the community to seek advice on adjusting your routine in response to life's curveballs.
- **Leverage Community Support:** Share your routine and progress with the Two Wolves community. This wolf pack provides a space for accountability, encouragement, and shared wisdom.
- **Reflect and Refine:** Regularly assess how your routine is serving you. Openly discuss with the wolf pack what's working and what isn't, allowing for collective insight to guide your adjustments.
- **Acknowledge Your Achievements:** Celebrate every step forward with the wolf pack. Acknowledging progress, both yours and others, fosters a positive environment and encourages continued effort.

Integrating these elements into your routine, with the active support of the Two Wolves community, not only propels you towards your personal goals but also reinforces the collective strength of the pack. Together, every member's success becomes a beacon of possibility, illuminating the path for others in their journey towards holistic wellness.

Daily Checklist (tick off)
□ Meditation
□ 10,000 Steps & Proof
□ Wolf Workout
□ Water Intake
□ 8-Hour Eating Window
□ Daily Learning (*Homework*)
□ Supplements (*Optional*)
□ 7+ Hours of Sleep
□ Daily Progress Photo
□ Alcohol & Sugar-Free

Reflecting on your current routine, what is one habit you recognize as detrimental to your well-being?

_____

_____

_____

_____

_____

How are you feeling today, and what role do you believe your current routine plays in influencing those feelings?

_____

_____

_____

_____

_____

_____

_____

_____

_____

_____

date ___ / ___ / ___

Journal the journey

Journal your thoughts on how you feel today and what steps you'll take to succeed tomorrow.

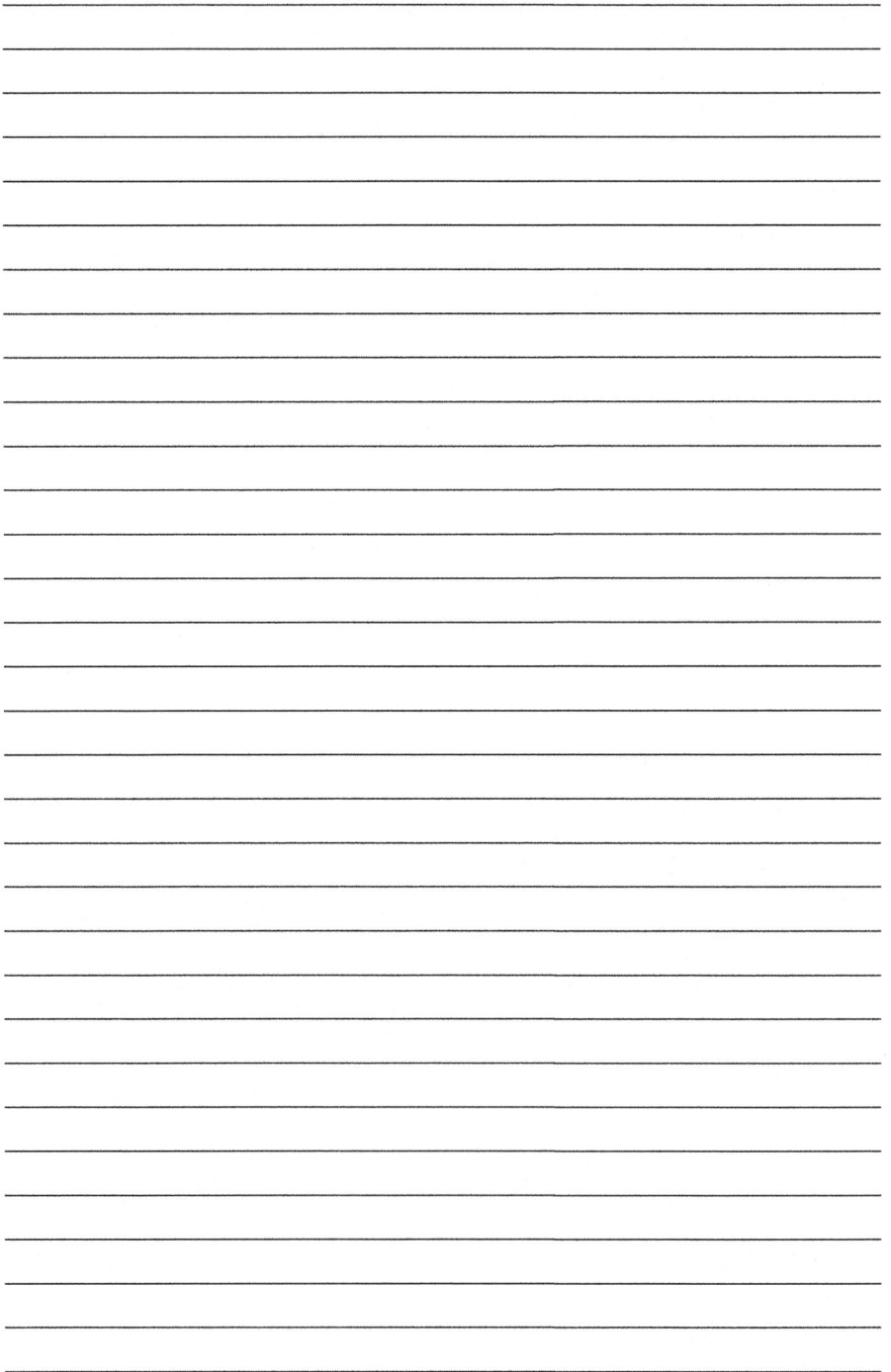

Day 6 Chapter 6
The power of sleep

"Sleep is the best meditation." – *Dalai Lama*

Sleep, often overlooked in the hustle of modern life, is the cornerstone of health and well-being. It's the time when the body embarks on its nightly journey of repair and renewal, a crucial process for maintaining physical and mental vigor. The Roman poet Ovid once said, *"Take rest; a field that has rested gives a bountiful crop."* This ancient wisdom echoes today's scientific understanding of sleep's indispensable role in our lives.

Scientific Insight into Sleep's Bounty
Extensive research underscores the transformative power of sleep. Studies, such as those published in the Journal of Sleep Research, have illuminated sleep's vital functions, from enhancing memory consolidation and cognitive performance to bolstering the immune system. Moreover, consistent quality sleep has been linked to reduced risks of chronic conditions such as obesity, type 2 diabetes, and heart disease. Conversely, the deprivation of sleep can sow seeds of stress, depression, and cognitive decline, underscoring the profound interconnection between sleep and our overall health landscape.

Crafting a Sanctuary for Sleep
Creating an environment conducive to sleep is paramount. This involves more than just physical comfort; it's about cultivating a haven for the mind and body. The environment should be serene—dark, quiet, and cool—to mimic the natural setting that signals our brain it's time for rest.

Additionally, aligning our sleep patterns with the circadian rhythm by adhering to regular sleep and wake times can significantly enhance sleep quality, as highlighted in research from the National Institute of Neurological Disorders and Stroke.

The Prelude to Slumber

The rituals we perform before bedtime play a critical role in easing the transition to sleep. A pre-sleep routine that might include reading, a warm bath, or meditation acts as a bridge from the day's busyness to the peaceful repose of night. Engaging in relaxation techniques before bed has been supported by studies like those in the Journal of Clinical Sleep Medicine, showing their efficacy in improving sleep quality.

Lifestyle's Embrace of Sleep

Our daily choices—what we eat, how we move, what we consume—intertwine closely with our sleep quality. Regular physical activity and a diet rich in nutrients lay the groundwork for restorative sleep, while it's wise to avoid stimulants like caffeine and disruptive elements like alcohol close to bedtime. The adage *"You are what you eat"* extends into *"Your sleep reflects how you live,"* a notion supported by extensive research including insights from the Sleep Health Journal.

Embracing Sleep's Embrace

To harness the power of sleep is to embrace a pillar of health as ancient as life itself. It's a commitment to nurturing the body's intrinsic need for restoration, a respect for the rhythm of existence that balances daylight's vigor with night's tranquility. As Shakespeare aptly noted in Macbeth, *"Sleep knits up the raveled sleeve of care..."* — a poetic testament to sleep's healing and fortifying essence.

Prioritizing sleep is akin to nurturing the soil from which the flowers of health and well-being bloom. By creating the right environment, engaging in conducive pre-sleep rituals, and adopting a lifestyle that honors our biological needs, we unlock the regenerative power of sleep. Let us, then, give ourselves to the night, trusting in the renewal that awaits with each dawn.

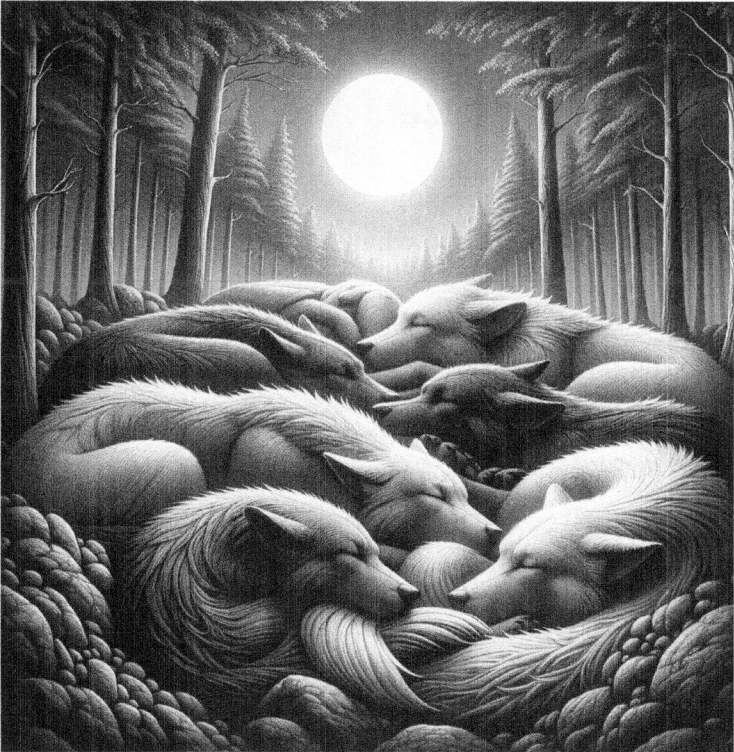

Daily Checklist (tick off)

☐ Meditation
☐ 10,000 Steps & Proof
☐ Wolf Workout
☐ Water Intake
☐ 8-Hour Eating Window
☐ Daily Learning (*Homework*)
☐ Supplements (*Optional*)
☐ 7+ Hours of Sleep
☐ Daily Progress Photo
☐ Alcohol & Sugar-Free

What aspect of your current sleep environment (darkness, noise, temperature) could most benefit from improvement, and what specific steps will you take to address this?

_____
_____
_____
_____
_____

How does your use of technology before bedtime currently impact your ability to fall asleep, and what strategy will you implement to minimize this effect?

_____
_____
_____
_____

How many hours of sleep do you typically get each night, and how do you feel upon waking? What actions could you take to either increase your sleep duration or enhance the quality of your rest?

_____
_____
_____

Journal the journey

Journal your thoughts on how you feel today and what steps you'll take to succeed tomorrow.

_____

_____

_____

_____

_____

_____

_____

_____

_____

_____

_____

_____

_____

_____

_____

_____

_____

_____

_____

_____

_____

_____

_____

_____

_____

_____

_____

_____

_____

_____

_____

_____

_____

_____

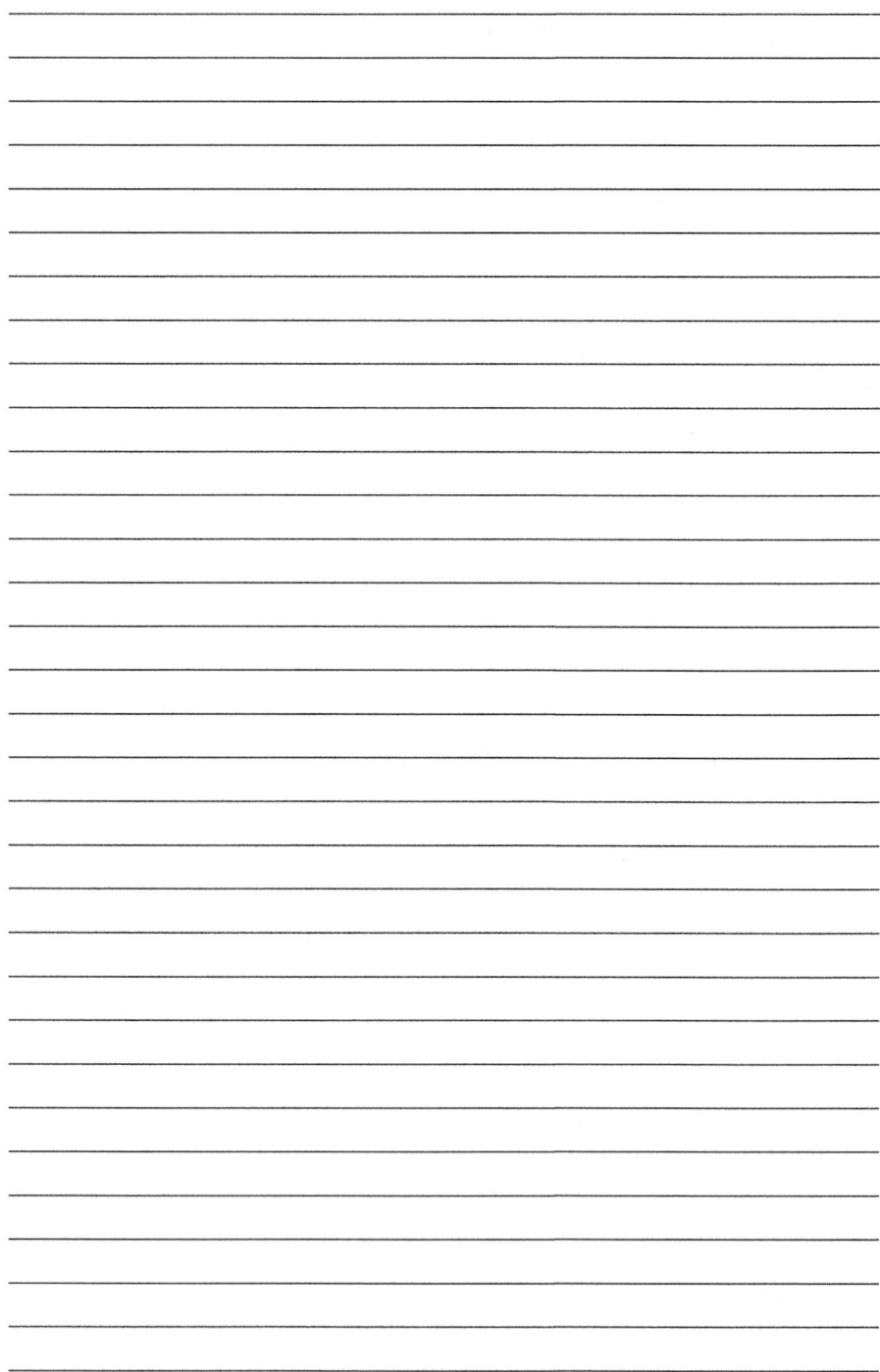

Day 7 Chapter 7
Cultivating Mindfulness

"Mindfulness isn't difficult, we just need to remember to do it."
– Sharon Salzberg

As you round off your first full week with the Two Wolves program, it's time to pause and appreciate your dedication. Successfully navigating the first seven days is no small feat; it marks the beginning of a profound transformation. However, with only a quarter of the journey behind us, we're poised to intensify our efforts. Now, let's channel even more energy into our workouts and delve deeper into the essence of mindfulness, a key tool in transcending heartbreak, procrastination, and negative thinking.

The Essence of Mindfulness

Mindfulness, the practice of maintaining a moment-by-moment awareness of our thoughts, feelings, bodily sensations, and the surrounding environment, is a beacon in navigating life's challenges. It's a skill that, when cultivated, offers a sanctuary of calm in the storm of our daily lives. Studies, such as those by Kabat-Zinn et al., have demonstrated that mindfulness meditation can significantly reduce symptoms of psychological stress, enhancing overall well-being.

Incorporating Mindfulness into Your Routine

Embedding mindfulness into your daily routine can transform mundane activities into moments of deep connection and insight. Start small—dedicate a few minutes each morning to sit in silence, focusing solely on your breath. This simple act can set a calm, centered tone for your day. Similarly, practice mindful eating by paying attention to the taste, texture, and sensations of your food, which can foster a healthier relationship with eating and curb mindless consumption.

Overcoming Adversity with Mindfulness

Heartbreak, procrastination, and negative thinking can deeply affect our well-being. Mindfulness offers a pathway out of these patterns. Engaging in heart-centered meditation, for example, can help process and heal emotional pain, as indicated by research in the Journal of Positive Psychology, which links mindfulness to greater emotional resilience. For procrastination, mindfulness strengthens our ability to focus and reduces the impulse to avoid challenging tasks, as suggested by studies in Consciousness and Cognition.

Practical Steps for Daily Mindfulness

- **Breathing Exercises:** Begin and end your day with a five-minute focused breathing exercise. This practice anchors your awareness in the present, helping to clear the mind of clutter and worry.
- **Mindful Movement:** Incorporate mindfulness into your Wolf Workout by concentrating on each movement and breath, turning exercise into a meditative practice.
- **Gratitude Journaling:** End each day by jotting down three things you're grateful for. This shifts focus from negative thinking to appreciation, enhancing emotional well-being.
- **Nature Walks:** Schedule regular walks in nature, using this time to observe the environment with all your senses. This connection to the natural world can heighten awareness and reduce feelings of stress.

The Path Forward

As we progress through the Two Wolves program, integrating mindfulness into our daily lives becomes not just a practice but a way of being. It empowers us to face life's adversities with grace and equanimity, fostering a deep inner strength that supports our journey towards holistic well-being. Remember, the mindful path is one of gentle persistence and open-hearted exploration. Embrace each moment with kindness and curiosity, and let mindfulness be your guide to a life of deeper fulfillment and joy.

Daily Checklist (tick off)

☐ Meditation
☐ 10,000 Steps & Proof
☐ Wolf Workout
☐ Water Intake
☐ 8-Hour Eating Window
☐ Daily Learning (*Homework*)
☐ Supplements (*Optional*)
☐ 7+ Hours of Sleep
☐ Daily Progress Photo
☐ Alcohol & Sugar-Free

How can incorporating a daily gratitude journaling practice transform your perspective on everyday challenges and successes?

_____
_____
_____
_____
_____

In what ways can mindful movement during your workouts deepen your connection to your physical and mental health goals?

_____
_____
_____
_____

What specific action will you take tomorrow to incorporate mindfulness into your routine?

_____
_____
_____
_____

Wolf Tracker 2

Congratulations on reaching an incredible milestone in your journey! You've been consistently pushing your limits for a whole week now, engaging with the Two Wolves program with dedication and courage. As you embark on the next phase, remember that growth occurs with each step you take, no matter how small. This week, it's time to revisit the Wolf Tracker 1 exercise and see how far you've come. Your perseverance is transforming potential into progress. Let's track your achievements and set new benchmarks!

Date: _____

Push Ups
- Week 1: _____
- Week 2: _____ (Record the number of push-ups you can perform in one minute.)

Squats
- Week 1: _____
- Week 2: _____ (Record the number of squats you can perform in one minute.)

Jumping Jacks
- Week 1: _____
- Week 2: _____ (Record the number of jumping jacks you can perform in one minute.)

Plank
- Week 1: _____
- Week 2: _____ (Record the duration you can hold the plank position.)

Reflect on your progress. Each number above represents more than just a count; it symbolizes your commitment, your growth, and the strength you're building every day. Use this moment to set new goals for the coming week, challenge yourself, and remember—the strength of the pack is within you.

Journal the journey

Journal your thoughts on how you feel today and what steps you'll take to succeed tomorrow.

_____
_____
_____
_____
_____
_____
_____
_____
_____
_____
_____
_____
_____
_____
_____
_____
_____
_____
_____
_____
_____
_____
_____
_____
_____
_____
_____
_____
_____
_____
_____
_____
_____
_____

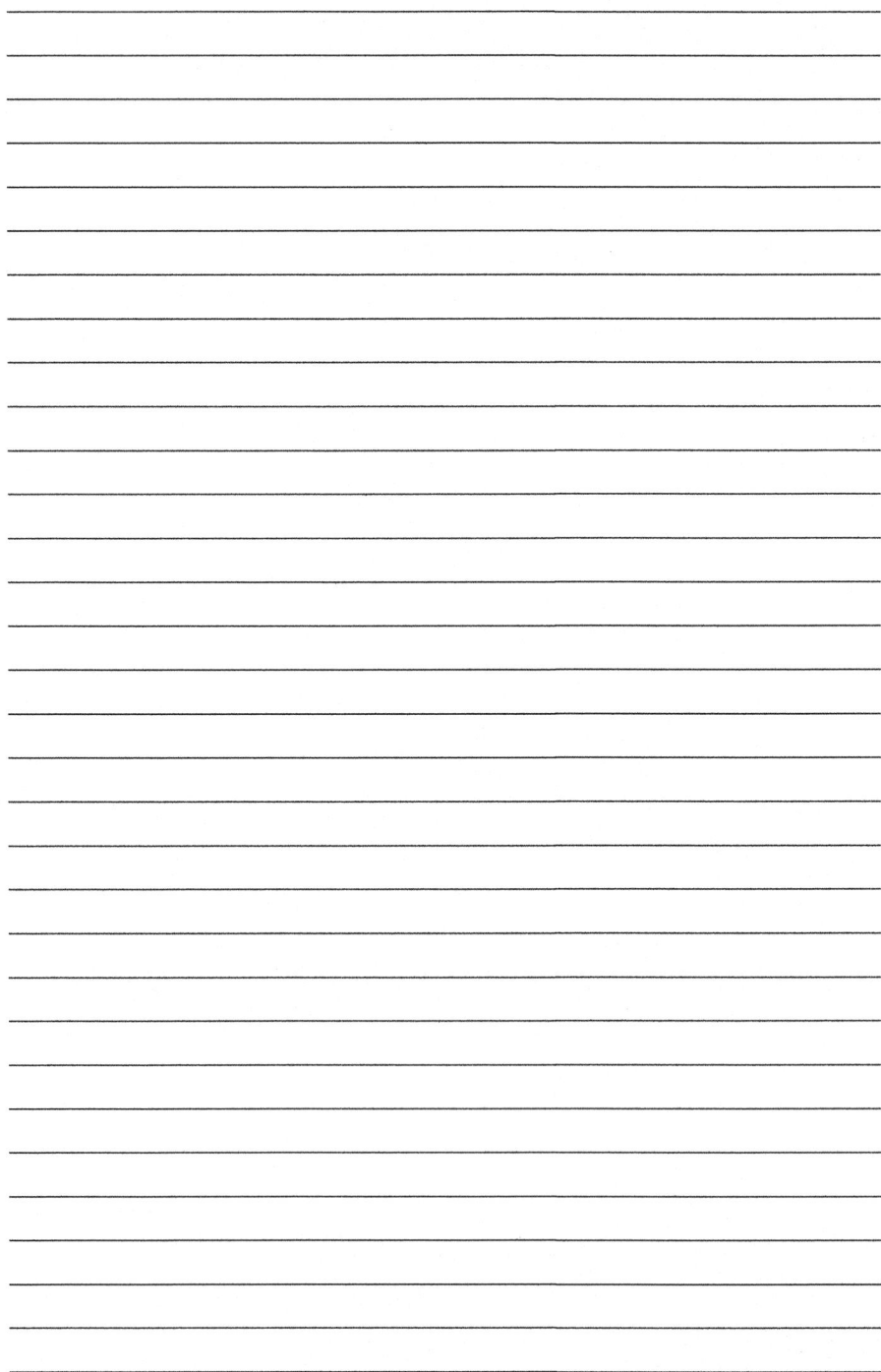

Wolf Workout Progression

Congratulations on completing Week 1 of your Wolf Workout journey! You've laid a solid foundation of strength and endurance, embracing the spirit of the wolf with every rep and set. As we step into Week 2, it's time to challenge ourselves further, introducing a progressive load to foster continued growth and improvement .

Here's your updated Wolf Workout for Week 2. This slight increase in reps and time is designed to push your boundaries safely and effectively, ensuring that you continue to progress on your path to strength and resilience.

- **Body Squats, Push-Ups, Leg Raises, and Step-Ups**: For each of these exercises, you'll perform 5 sets of **6 repetitions**. This increase from 5 reps ensures a gradual intensification of your workout, promoting muscle growth and endurance without overburdening your body.

- **Elbow Plank**: Extend your plank hold to **35 seconds** per set. This additional time continues to challenge your core, enhancing stability and strength.

As you embark on Week 2, remember the lessons of the two wolves: the growth and progress you feed are the ones that flourish. Embrace this week's challenge with determination and mindfulness, listening to your body and respecting its limits while pushing towards greater achievements.

Each exercise in this program is a step towards unleashing your inner wolf and building a stronger, more resilient version of yourself. Stay committed, stay motivated, and let the spirit of the wolf guide you through this week's journey.

Phase II

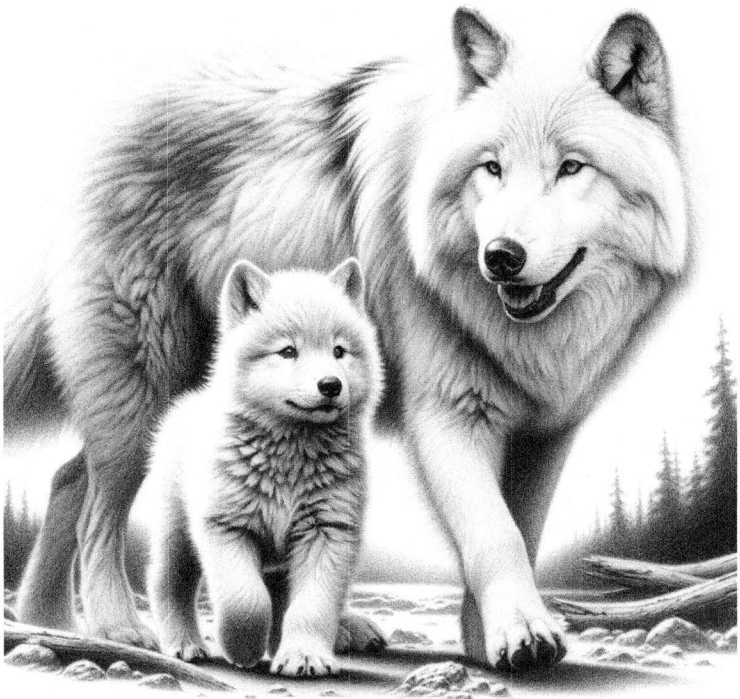

Trasnsformations

Day 8 Chapter 8
Goal Setting

"The greater danger for most of us lies not in setting our aim too high and falling short; but in setting our aim too low, and achieving our mark." - *Michelangelo*

The Philosophical and Historical Context of Goal-Setting
The practice of setting goals is not merely a modern phenomenon but a timeless aspect of human experience, deeply embedded in both Western and Eastern philosophical traditions. In the West, the Stoic philosophers, such as Marcus Aurelius and Seneca, emphasized the importance of living a life guided by reason and virtue, advocating for setting goals aligned with one's nature and the common good. They believed that a well-lived life is the result of deliberate intention and purposeful action, echoing the sentiment that "*Luck is what happens when preparation meets opportunity*" (Seneca).

Similarly, Eastern philosophies, including Buddhism and Taoism, place a strong emphasis on intention, mindfulness, and the journey towards enlightenment. The Buddhist concept of "Right Intention," one of the steps in the Noble Eightfold Path, encourages setting goals that promote harmony, peace, and compassion towards oneself and others. These ancient teachings underscore the universal recognition of goal-setting as a crucial element in the pursuit of personal and collective well-being.

Scientific Perspectives on Goal-Setting
Turning to the realm of psychology, the Goal-Setting Theory developed by Locke and Latham provides a robust framework for understanding the motivational power of goals.

Their research elucidates how specific and challenging goals enhance performance by directing focus, mobilizing effort, and promoting persistence. Moreover, neuroscience studies have begun to uncover the neural mechanisms underpinning goal-directed behaviors, demonstrating the role of the prefrontal cortex in goal formulation and the dopamine system in motivation and reward. These findings from cognitive science and behavioral psychology affirm the efficacy of goal-setting as a catalyst for personal achievement and self-improvement.

Formulating Effective Goals: Beyond the Basics
While the SMART criteria lay the groundwork for effective goal-setting, true mastery involves a deeper engagement with one's goals. It requires introspection to ensure that your goals resonate with your core values and life's purpose. Reflect on what brings you joy, fulfillment, and a sense of accomplishment. Incorporate these insights into your goals to ensure they are deeply meaningful and motivating.

Additionally, the process of goal-setting should be dynamic and adaptive. Life's inevitable changes and challenges may necessitate revising your goals. Cultivate flexibility in your approach, allowing your goals to evolve in alignment with your growth and experiences. Regular reflection and adjustment ensure your goals remain relevant and impactful.

The Psychological and Philosophical Dimensions of Goal-Setting
Understanding the psychological underpinnings of goal-setting can enhance its effectiveness. Engage with cognitive-behavioral strategies to overcome barriers such as procrastination and fear of failure. Techniques such as positive self-talk, visualization, and incremental goal-setting can build confidence and momentum. Philosophically, consider the concept of "Eudaimonia," a term from Aristotelian ethics representing the condition of human flourishing or living well.

Your goals should contribute to a life of eudaimonia, reflecting a harmonious balance between duty, personal growth, and the pursuit of happiness.

The Journey Is the Goal: The Process of Becoming
Ultimately, goal-setting is about the journey as much as the destination. It is a process of continuous learning, growth, and self-discovery. Embrace each step of the journey, celebrating progress and learning from setbacks. The path toward achieving your goals is rich with opportunities for developing resilience, cultivating wisdom, and deepening your understanding of yourself and the world around you.

Goal-setting is a profound and multi-faceted practice, bridging ancient philosophical insights with modern scientific understanding. It is an art and science of envisioning a desired future and systematically working towards it, embodying the principles of intentionality, self-awareness, and perseverance. By embracing the depth and complexity of goal-setting, you can unlock your potential and embark on a transformative journey toward personal excellence and fulfillment.

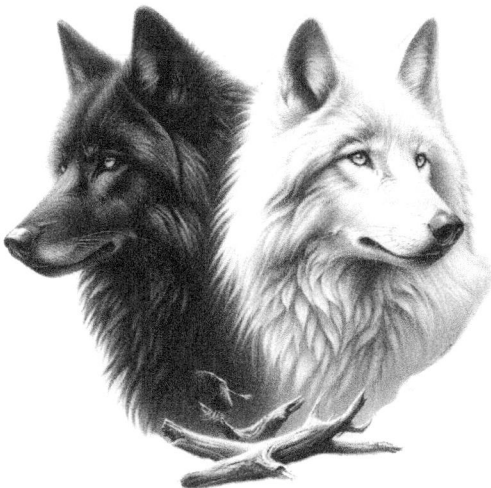

Daily Checklist (tick off)
☐ Meditation
☐ 10,000 Steps & Proof
☐ Wolf Workout
☐ Water Intake
☐ 8-Hour Eating Window
☐ Daily Learning (*Homework*)
☐ Supplements (*Optional*)
☐ 7+ Hours of Sleep
☐ Daily Progress Photo
☐ Alcohol & Sugar-Free

Consider a goal you've struggled to achieve in the past. Identify the main obstacles that hindered your progress. How can you approach these challenges differently this time to ensure success?

_____
_____
_____
_____
_____

Complete a focused task or project you've been postponing, breaking it down into smaller, manageable steps. what is it?

._____
_____
_____
_____
_____

What specific goal do you aim to achieve by the end of this 30-day challenge that will significantly improve your well-being or lifestyle?

_____
_____
_____
_____

date ___ / ___ / ___

Journal the journey

Journal your thoughts on how you feel today and what steps you'll take to succeed tomorrow.

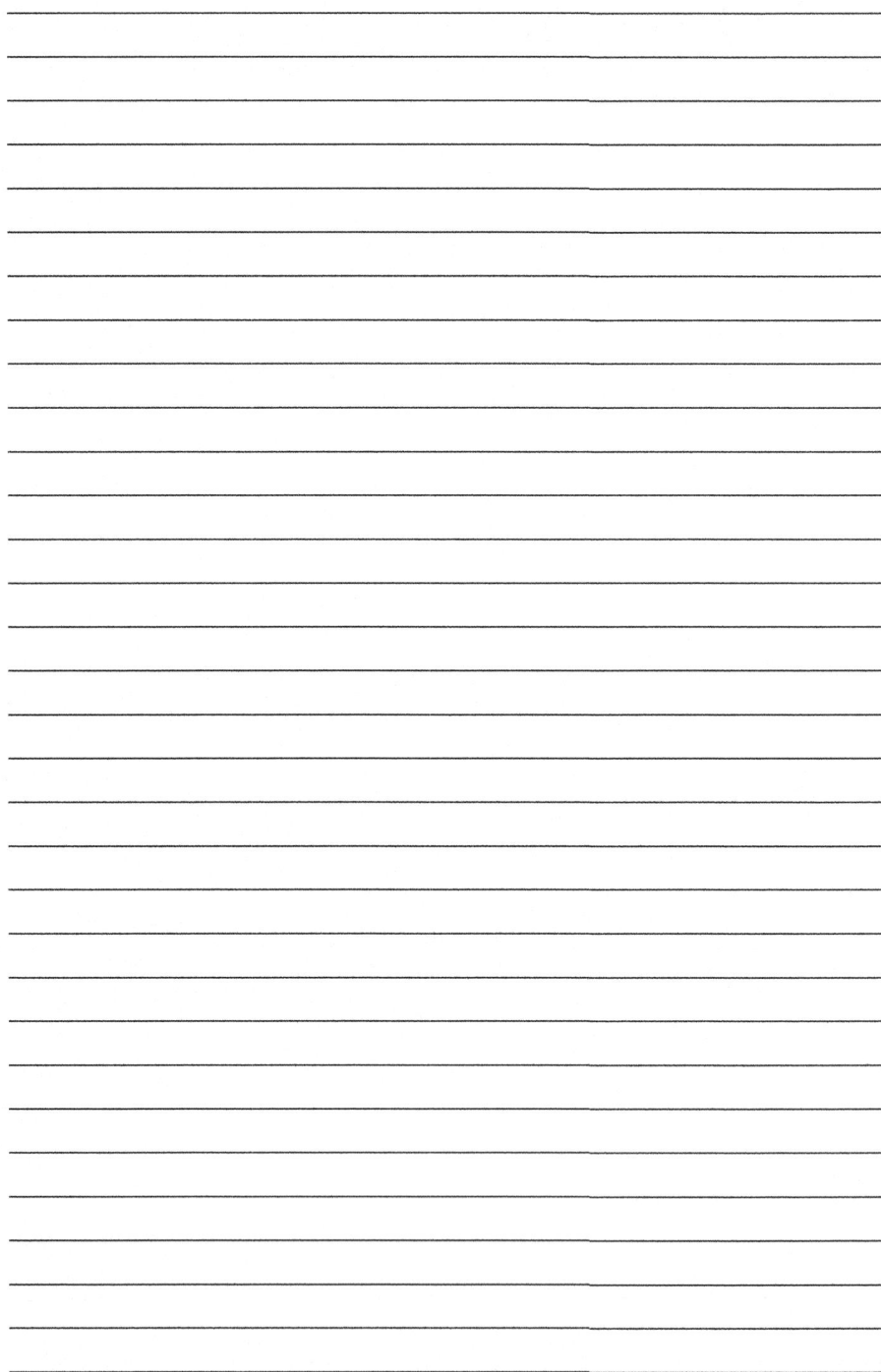

Day 9 Chapter 9
Maximise Motivation

"The greatest glory in living lies not in never falling, but in rising every time we fall." - *Nelson Mandela*

Motivation, the vital energy that propels us toward our aspirations, acts as the catalyst for change and achievement. Yet, its presence often ebbs and flows, leaving many in search of ways to reignite that inner spark. This chapter delves into the art and science of sustaining high levels of motivation, drawing upon timeless wisdom and cutting-edge research to guide you in awakening your inner wolf—the embodiment of determination, resilience, and focus.

Understanding the nature of motivation is crucial; it is inherently dynamic, subject to the natural rhythms of human psychology and physiology. Accepting this variability is the first step toward harnessing motivation more effectively. As the Roman philosopher Seneca wisely articulated, "*It is not because things are difficult that we do not dare; it is because we do not dare that they are difficult.*" This ancient insight reminds us that our perception and attitude toward challenges significantly influence our motivational drive.

Setting precise, tangible goals is a foundational strategy for fostering motivation. Goals act as the north star, guiding our efforts and providing a measurable framework for progress. The power of goal-setting is well-documented in contemporary research, with studies demonstrating its positive impact on performance and achievement. To make the most of this strategy, break down overarching objectives into smaller, manageable tasks. Celebrating each minor victory fuels your motivation, creating a positive feedback loop that propels you toward your ultimate target.

The significance of mindset in sustaining motivation cannot be overstated. The concept of "growth mindset," popularized by psychologist Carol Dweck, emphasizes the belief in our ability to develop and improve through effort and persistence. This perspective encourages resilience in the face of adversity, a critical component of sustained motivation. By embracing challenges as opportunities for growth, you cultivate an indomitable spirit that thrives on progress.

Support systems play a pivotal role in nurturing motivation. Surrounding yourself with a community of supportive peers and mentors creates an environment conducive to growth and accountability. As Aristotle famously noted, *"The whole is greater than the sum of its parts."* This ancient wisdom highlights the exponential power of collective support in achieving personal goals. Prioritizing physical and mental health is equally essential for maintaining motivation. Research underscores the interconnectivity between physical activity, nutrition, and mental well-being in influencing our energy levels and motivational states. Regular exercise, a balanced diet, and adequate rest are fundamental to optimizing your body and mind for peak performance. Additionally, mindfulness practices such as meditation can significantly reduce stress levels, enhancing your capacity to focus and remain motivated.

In summary, maximizing motivation is a multifaceted endeavor that requires a harmonious blend of strategic goal-setting, a resilient mindset, robust support networks, and a commitment to physical and mental health. By integrating these principles, rooted in both ancient wisdom and modern science, you can ignite your inner wolf's spirit, embarking on a path of purposeful action and extraordinary achievement.

To effectively apply the insights from this chapter to your challenge, consider integrating the following tips into your daily routine:

- **Define Your Why:** Start by clarifying your purpose for taking on this challenge. Understanding your "why" will serve as your anchor, keeping you motivated even when the journey gets tough.
- **Set Specific Goals:** Break down your 30-day challenge into smaller, actionable goals. For instance, if your challenge includes improving physical fitness, set weekly targets for exercise intensity or duration. Document these goals and your progress toward them.
- **Cultivate a Growth Mindset:** Embrace challenges as opportunities for growth. When you encounter obstacles, remind yourself of Carol Dweck's growth mindset principle and view these moments as chances to learn and improve.
- **Build a Support System:** Engage actively with the Two Wolves Facebook community. Share your goals, seek advice, and offer support to others. The encouragement and accountability from this community can be a powerful motivator.
- **Incorporate Mindfulness Practices:** Dedicate time each day for mindfulness or meditation, aiming to increase your awareness and presence. This practice can help reduce stress and enhance your focus, contributing positively to your motivation.
- **Maintain Physical Well-being:** Prioritize exercise, nutritious eating, and sufficient sleep. These physical aspects significantly impact your energy levels and motivation, enabling you to perform your best throughout the challenge.
- **Celebrate Progress:** Acknowledge and celebrate your achievements, no matter how small. These celebrations reinforce your progress and keep the motivational fire burning.

- **Reflect and Adjust:** Regularly reflect on your experience and the strategies you're using. Are they working for you? If not, don't hesitate to adjust your approach based on what you've learned about maintaining motivation.

By thoughtfully applying these tips, you'll be better equipped to maintain high levels of motivation throughout the challenge, bringing you closer to achieving your personal growth and development goals.

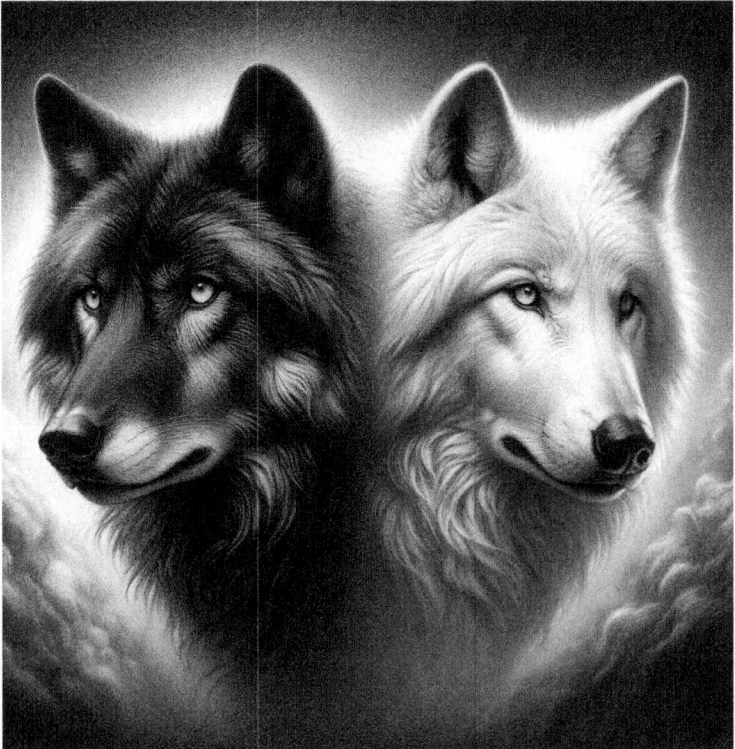

Daily Checklist (tick off)

☐ Meditation
☐ 10,000 Steps & Proof
☐ Wolf Workout
☐ Water Intake
☐ 8-Hour Eating Window
☐ Daily Learning (*Homework*)
☐ Supplements (*Optional*)
☐ 7+ Hours of Sleep
☐ Daily Progress Photo
☐ Alcohol & Sugar-Free

What's one small goal you can set for tomorrow to boost your motivation?

_____
_____
_____
_____
_____

How will you remind yourself of your "why" each day this week?

_____
_____
_____
_____

What's one way you can reward yourself for meeting a daily goal to stay motivated?

_____
_____
_____
_____

Journal the journey

Journal your thoughts on how you feel today and what steps you'll take to succeed tomorrow.

_____

_____

_____

_____

_____

_____

_____

_____

_____

_____

_____

_____

_____

_____

_____

_____

_____

_____

_____

_____

_____

_____

_____

_____

_____

_____

_____

_____

_____

_____

_____

_____

_____

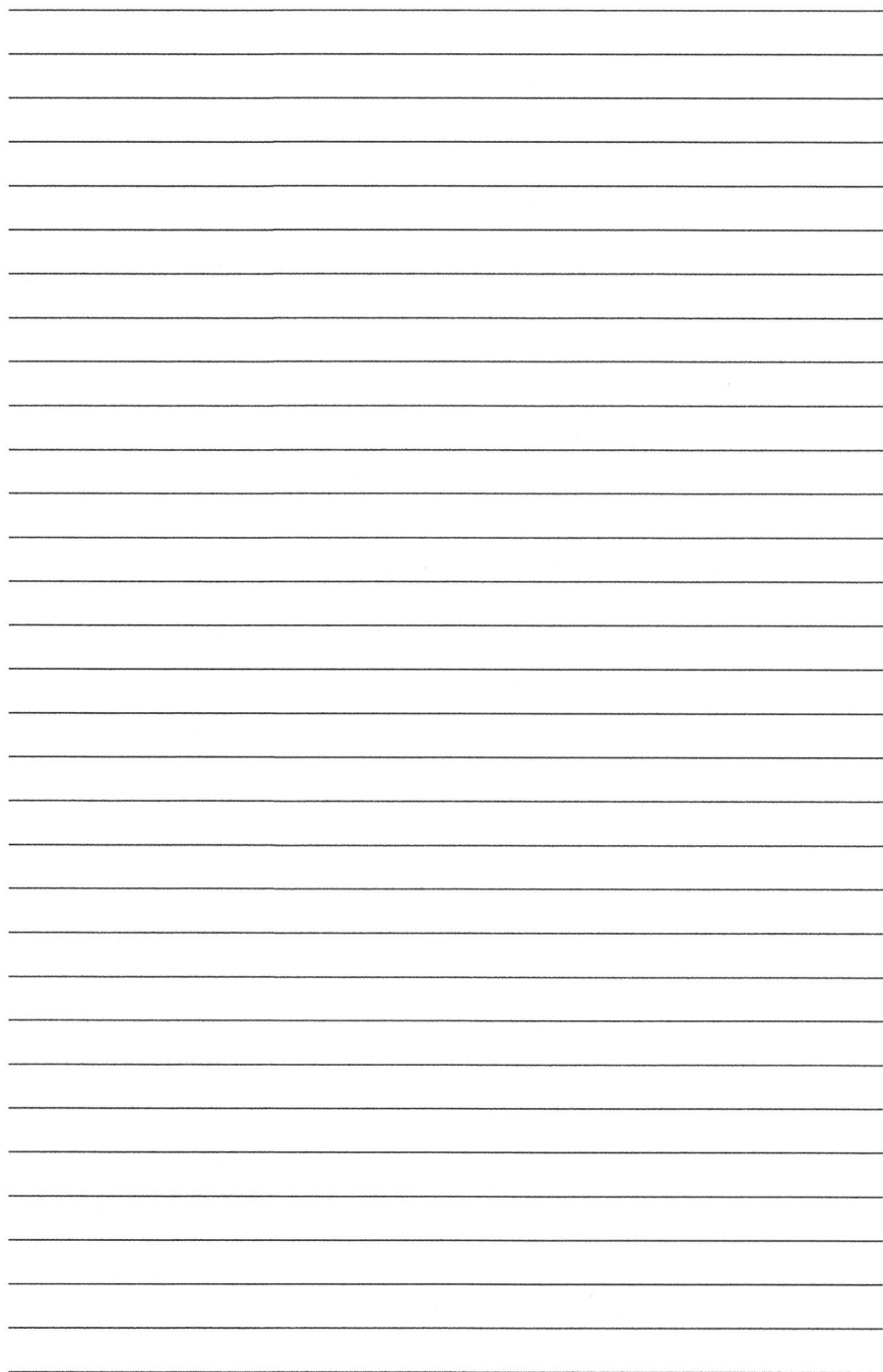

Day 10 Chapter 10
Pushing Past Plateaus

"Continuous effort - not strength or intelligence - is the key to unlocking our potential." - Winston Churchill

Experiencing a fitness plateau can feel like hitting an invisible wall. Your dedication and hard work suddenly seem to yield no further progress, transforming motivation into a test of perseverance. It's essential to recognize that these plateaus are not dead ends but rather integral milestones in your fitness journey. As we approach Day 10, you might encounter your first plateau; this is not a signal to surrender but an opportunity to recalibrate and surge forward.

Plateaus in fitness are often misunderstood. They're not markers of failure but signs of your body's remarkable adaptability. The stagnation in progress—whether it's in weight loss, muscle gain, or endurance—signals it's time for change. This phase, encountered by countless athletes and fitness enthusiasts, is where innovation meets determination.

Incorporating Diversity in Your Routine

The key to overcoming plateaus lies in variation. Our bodies thrive on challenge and novelty. Introducing new exercises or altering your workout's intensity, duration, and frequency can reignite progress. Science supports the efficacy of this approach. A study in the Journal of Strength and Conditioning Research highlights how altering workout routines every two weeks significantly enhances strength and endurance over a 10-week period.

Celebrating Your Journey

Shift your focus from what's pending to the milestones you've already achieved.

A mindset anchored in gratitude amplifies resilience and determination. Consider maintaining a fitness journal, not just for tracking workouts and nutrition, but for acknowledging daily victories, no matter their size.

Prioritizing Recovery
Often overlooked, recovery is paramount. Your progress hinges on how well you rest and recuperate. Overtraining can lead to injuries and burnout, halting progress entirely. Embrace rest days with the same enthusiasm as workout days, ensuring adequate sleep and proper nutrition. This holistic approach fosters both physical and mental rejuvenation, preparing you for greater challenges ahead.

Maintaining a Growth Mindset
Renowned psychologist Carol Dweck's work on growth mindset unveils the power of perspective. Viewing plateaus as learning curves rather than obstacles can transform them into powerful motivators. As you encounter these plateaus, ask yourself, "What can I learn from this?" rather than "Why am I stuck?" In essence, fitness plateaus are not just hurdles to overcome but crucial aspects of your growth story. They prompt you to explore new territories, refine your strategies, and deepen your commitment to your health and fitness aspirations. With the right mindset, varied routine, and balanced recovery, you'll not only transcend these plateaus but emerge stronger, wiser, and more capable than ever before.

"Do not pray for an easy life, pray for the strength to endure a difficult one." - Bruce Lee

This journey you're on is about forging a version of yourself that thrives on challenge, celebrates every step of progress, and recognizes the power of resilience. As we move forward, let's embrace each plateau not as a barrier but as a gateway to newfound strengths and possibilities.

Daily Checklist (tick off)

☐ Meditation

☐ 10,000 Steps & Proof

☐ Wolf Workout

☐ Water Intake

☐ 8-Hour Eating Window

☐ Daily Learning (*Homework*)

☐ Supplements (*Optional*)

☐ 7+ Hours of Sleep

☐ Daily Progress Photo

☐ Alcohol & Sugar-Free

What new exercise or activity can you introduce into your routine this week to challenge your body in a new way?

_____

_____

_____

_____

_____

Reflecting on your journey so far, what are three achievements or aspects of your progress you're grateful for?

_____

_____

_____

_____

_____

What small adjustment can you make to your current workout intensity or duration to push past a plateau?

_____

_____

_____

_____

Journal the journey

Journal your thoughts on how you feel today and what steps you'll take to succeed tomorrow.

_____

_____

_____

_____

_____

_____

_____

_____

_____

_____

_____

_____

_____

_____

_____

_____

_____

_____

_____

_____

_____

_____

_____

_____

_____

_____

_____

_____

_____

_____

_____

_____

_____

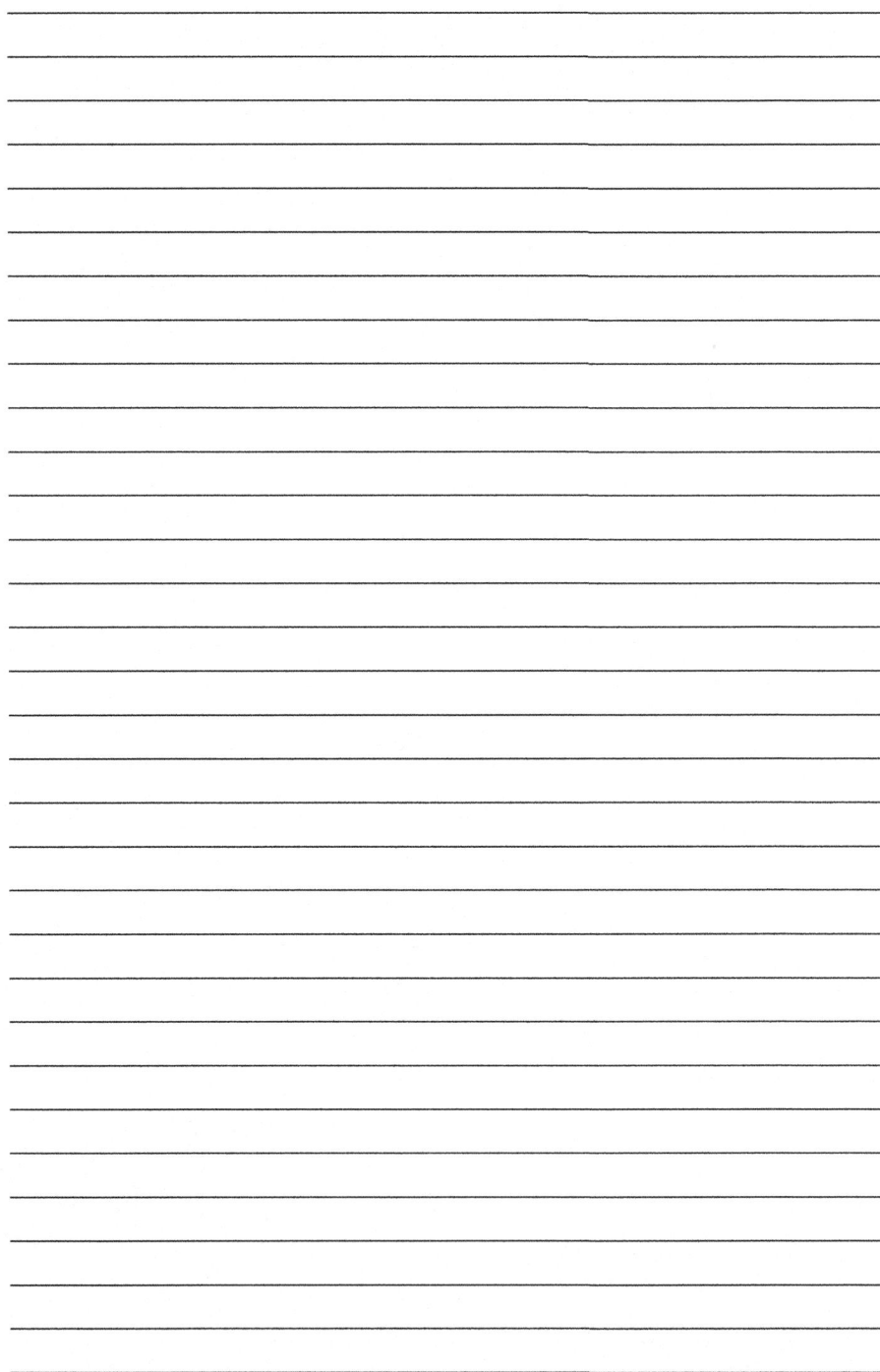

Day 11 Chapter 11
Falling from the Pack

""There are two types of people in this world: those who say they can and those who say they can't. They're both right." - *Henry Ford*

In life's marathon, it's inevitable we sometimes falter, trailing behind our envisioned pace. The moments when our stride falters, missing the targeted 10,000 steps or a day's workout, can feel like a solitary fall from the collective pursuit of progress. This juncture, seemingly cloaked in setback, invites a profound question: What unfolds when we diverge from the pack's rhythm? Far from a mere lapse, these moments herald a potent brew of introspection and growth.

Ancient wisdom reminds us that every detour is a path laden with lessons. Lao Tzu once mused, *"A journey of a thousand miles begins with a single step."* But what of the steps that stray? They too are integral to our journey, carving paths to unexplored terrains within ourselves.

Science echoes this, illustrating that setbacks, far from ending journeys, enrich them. Psychological resilience, a concept widely studied, underscores the elasticity of the human spirit. Research in the "Journal of Behavioral Medicine" illuminates how challenges, including physical and motivational lapses, can fortify our mental resilience, teaching us to navigate the undulating terrains of life and ambition with grace.

Falling behind is not a cessation but a pause, an opportunity to recalibrate our compass. Revisiting our aspirations, we ponder: Are these pursuits true reflections of our inner fire?

Adjusting our lens to focus on intrinsic motivation can rekindle the embers of commitment, guiding us back with renewed vigor.

The camaraderie of the pack, too, plays a vital role. As Helen Keller insightfully put it, *"Alone we can do so little; together we can do so much."* The community's wisdom, the collective 'Den,' serves as both a sanctuary and a beacon, propelling us forward through shared strength and encouragement.

Moreover, this juncture might beckon us towards uncharted territories in our fitness odyssey. Innovation, the willingness to infuse our routine with fresh vigor—whether through new exercises, environments, or challenges—can illuminate undiscovered facets of our resilience and capability.

In traversing the vast landscape of life and aspiration, detours are not merely obstacles but gateways to deeper understanding and growth. They remind us that the essence of our journey lies not in unwavering adherence to the pack but in the courage to embrace our unique rhythm, supported by the unwavering spirit of the pack. As we weave through the tapestry of trials and triumphs, we emerge not just participants in the race but as architects of our own extraordinary odyssey. We are the pack, and in unity, we find our strength to surmount any divergence and reach the finish line, together.

Actionable Advice

- **Reconnect with Your 'Why':** When you find yourself lagging, revisit the core reason you started this journey. Your 'why' is a powerful motivator that can help you push through challenging moments.
- **Lean on the Pack:** Utilize the Two Wolves community 'Den' for support and motivation. Sharing your struggles and victories with others who understand can provide a boost of encouragement and remind you that you're not alone.

- **Celebrate Every Success:** No victory is too small. Celebrated achievements, no matter their size, fuel your motivation and highlight your progress, keeping you engaged and focused.
- **Incorporate Mindfulness into Your Routine:** Practicing mindfulness can enhance your connection with the present moment, reducing stress and amplifying your focus on your goals. Try starting or ending your day with a few minutes of meditation to center your mind.
- **Visualize Your Success:** Spend time each day visualizing achieving your goals. This mental rehearsal can boost your confidence and motivation, making your goals feel more attainable.
- **Stay Committed to Daily Habits:** Adherence to your daily tasks, such as meditation, the Wolf Workout, and the 10,000 steps, is crucial. Consistency in these habits builds momentum and fosters a sense of accomplishment.
- **Adjust Your Perspective on Setbacks:** View any setbacks not as failures but as learning opportunities. Understanding what led to the setback can be enlightening and guide you to strengthen your approach moving forward.
- **Engage in Positive Self-Talk:** Replace negative thoughts with positive affirmations. Reminding yourself of your strength, resilience, and capability can help maintain your motivation.
- **Ensure Proper Rest and Recovery**: Recognizing the importance of rest, ensure you're getting adequate sleep and using relaxation techniques to recover fully, enabling you to tackle each day's tasks with renewed energy.
- **Stay Hydrated and Nourish Your Body:** Proper hydration and nutrition are key components of your fitness journey. They support your physical health, energy levels, and overall well-being, contributing to your ability to stay motivated and focused.

Daily Checklist (tick off)

☐ Meditation

☐ 10,000 Steps & Proof

☐ Wolf Workout

☐ Water Intake

☐ 8-Hour Eating Window

☐ Daily Learning (*Homework*)

☐ Supplements (*Optional*)

☐ 7+ Hours of Sleep

☐ Daily Progress Photo

☐ Alcohol & Sugar-Free

What is one positive affirmation you can tell yourself during challenging moments to maintain a positive mindset?

_____

_____

_____

_____

_____

How will you practice self-compassion today if you feel like you're falling behind, reminding yourself that progress, not perfection, is the goal?

._____

_____

_____

_____

_____

In what ways can you celebrate your progress so far, even the small victories, to maintain momentum?

_____

_____

_____

_____

date ___ / ___ / ___

Journal the journey

Journal your thoughts on how you feel today and what steps you'll take to succeed tomorrow.

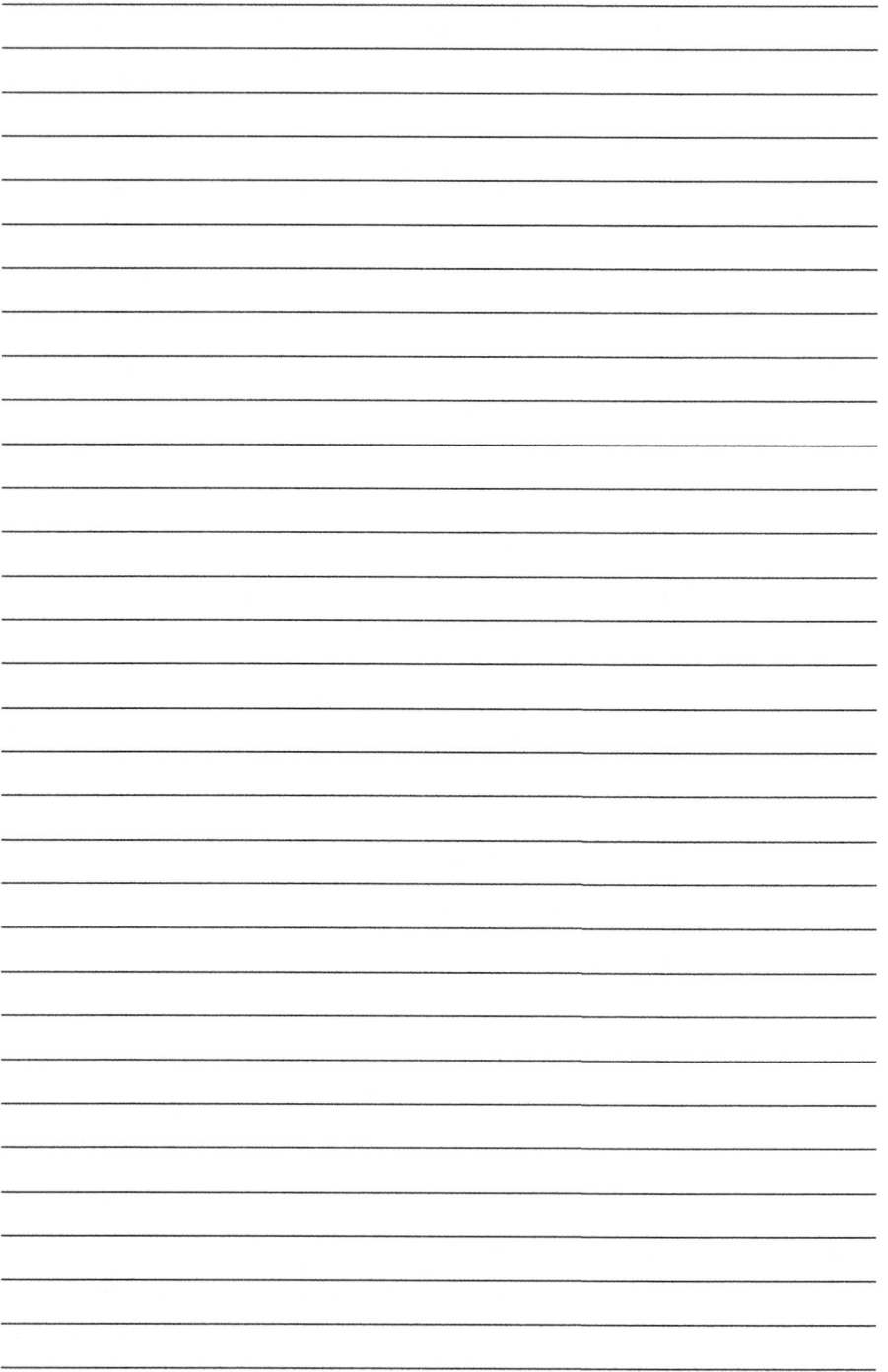

Day 12 Chapter 12
Accountability & You

"Continuous effort - not strength or intelligence - is the key to unlocking our potential."
- *Winston Churchill*

In the quest for personal and professional growth, accountability stands as a beacon, guiding us through the challenges and toward our aspirations. It's the silent pact we make with ourselves and others, a commitment to pursue our goals relentlessly. This chapter delves into the essence of accountability, unraveling its significance and offering actionable strategies to harness its power.

Understanding Accountability
Accountability transcends mere responsibility; it's an introspective journey where we align our actions with our deepest values and intentions. It means not only celebrating our victories but also owning our setbacks, understanding that each step—forward or backward—is part of the path to success. Ancient wisdom, like the teachings of Stoicism, emphasizes control over one's own actions and reactions, a principle mirrored in modern accountability practices.

Setting Specific, Measurable Goals
The first step to enhancing accountability is through goal specificity. The ancient philosopher Seneca's advice, "*If one does not know to which port one is sailing, no wind is favorable,*" echoes the importance of clear, targeted goals. Modern studies support this, showing that specific and challenging goals lead to higher performance (Locke & Latham, 2002). By dissecting ambitious aspirations into tangible, achievable milestones, we create a roadmap for success, allowing for periodic reflection and course correction.

Enlisting Support

No wolf pack thrives in isolation, and neither do we. Enlisting the support of peers, mentors, or coaches not only provides a motivational boost but also introduces diverse perspectives and insights. This collaborative approach, grounded in ancient tribal societies' emphasis on communal success, is bolstered by modern research indicating that social support is critical in achieving and maintaining goal-directed behaviors (Carron, Hausenblas, & Estabrooks, 2003).

Cultivating Self-Discipline

At its core, accountability is deeply personal. It's about developing the self-discipline to adhere to our commitments when no one else is watching. Drawing on the wisdom of Marcus Aurelius, "Such as your habitual thoughts, such also will be the character of your mind; for the soul is dyed by the thoughts," we see the importance of nurturing a mindset oriented toward discipline and self-improvement.

Embracing Feedback

True growth occurs at the intersection of effort and receptivity to feedback. Constructive criticism, though often challenging to accept, is a crucible for development. It echoes the teachings of Socrates on the value of inquiry and reflection in the pursuit of wisdom. Modern psychological research underscores the importance of feedback in adjusting strategies and behaviors toward goal achievement (Hattie & Timperley, 2007).

Actionable Tips to Implement Accountability
- **Daily Reflections:** Dedicate time each day to reflect on your progress, challenges, and the steps needed to move closer to your goals.

- **Accountability Partners:** Pair up with someone who shares similar goals. Regularly update each other on your progress and hurdles.
- **Public Commitment:** Share your goals with a wider circle to increase your sense of commitment and receive broad-based support.
- **Set Up Reminders:** Use technology to set reminders for your goals, reflecting on ancient principles of regular, mindful practice.
- **Reward System:** Create a system of rewards for milestones achieved, tapping into the human propensity for positive reinforcement.

Accountability is not a burden but a liberation. It frees us from the confines of aimlessness and propels us toward our highest potential. Like the wolf who thrives within the structure and support of the pack, we too can harness the power of accountability to navigate the wilderness of our aspirations and emerge triumphant.

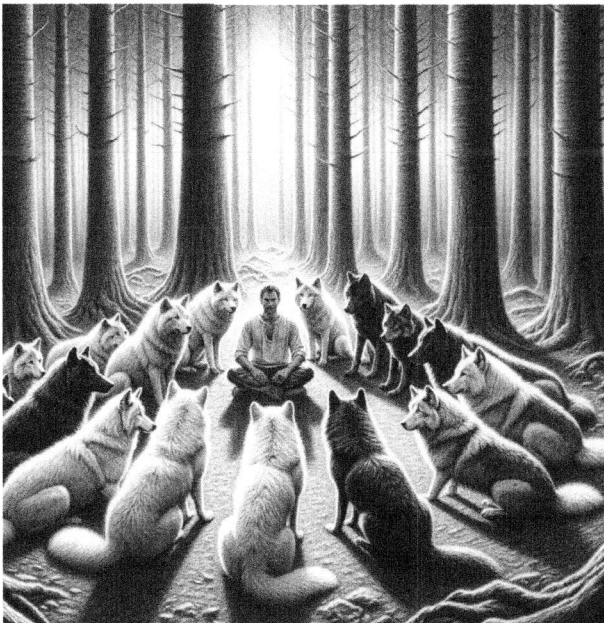

Daily Checklist (tick off)

☐ Meditation
☐ 10,000 Steps & Proof
☐ Wolf Workout
☐ Water Intake
☐ 8-Hour Eating Window
☐ Daily Learning (*Homework*)
☐ Supplements (*Optional*)
☐ 7+ Hours of Sleep
☐ Daily Progress Photo
☐ Alcohol & Sugar-Free

Who will you choose as your accountability partner to share your journey and goals with?

_____

_____

_____

_____

_____

In what area of your life do you need to take more responsibility, and how will you start?

_____

_____

_____

_____

_____

How will you respond to feedback or criticism to improve yourself?

_____

_____

_____

_____

date _____ / ___ / _____

Journal the journey

Journal your thoughts on how you feel today and what steps you'll take to succeed tomorrow.

_____

_____
_____
_____
_____
_____
_____
_____
_____
_____
_____
_____
_____
_____
_____
_____
_____
_____
_____
_____
_____
_____
_____
_____
_____
_____
_____
_____
_____
_____
_____
_____
_____
_____

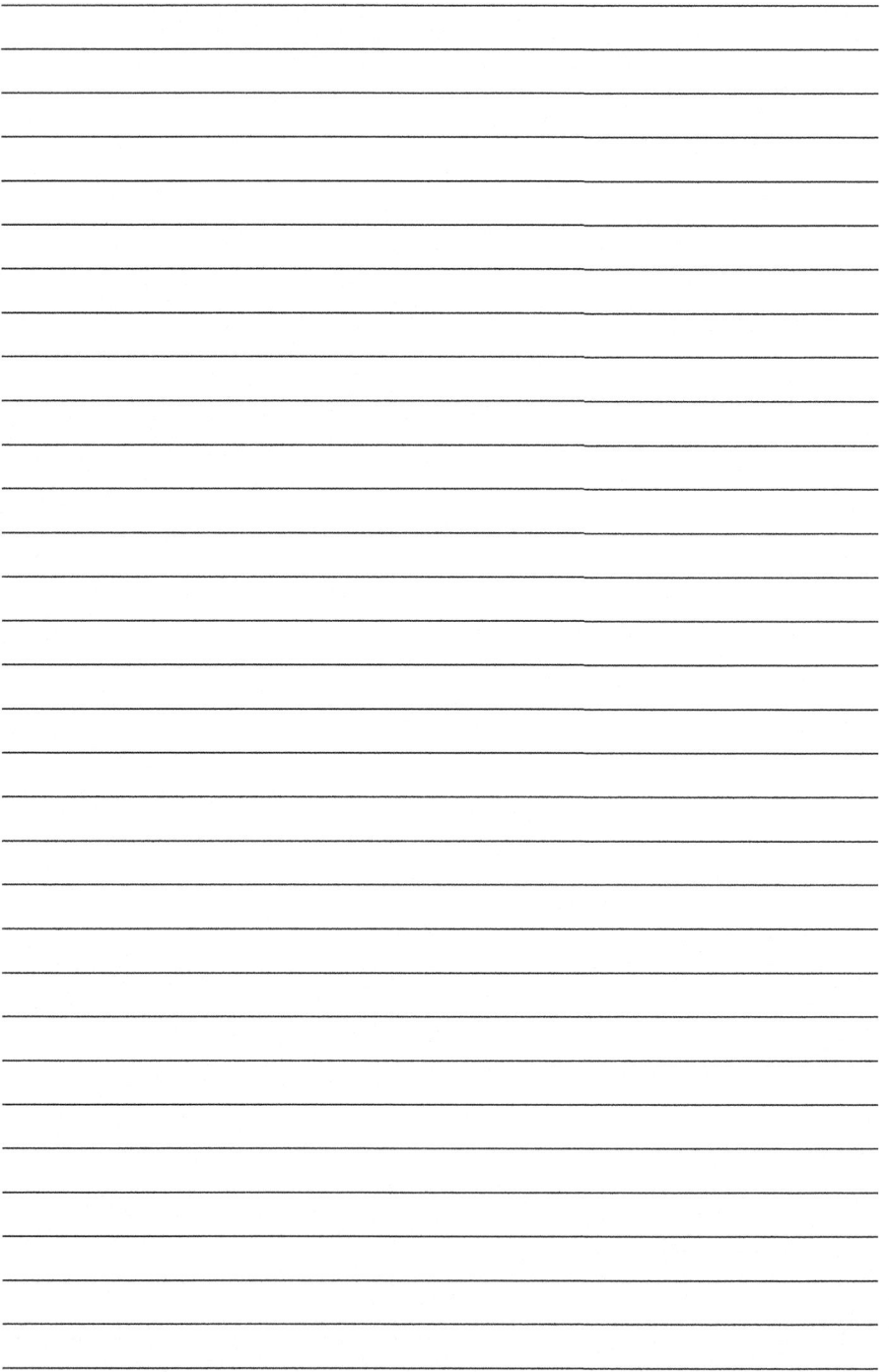

Day 13 Chapter 13
Progress & Wins

"Without deviation from the norm, progress is not possible."
-Frank Zappa

The pursuit of personal growth is akin to navigating a vast and uncharted terrain. It demands resilience, patience, and an unwavering focus, reminding us that progress is not solely about reaching a distant peak but cherishing each stride that brings us closer to our summit. In this narrative of self-discovery, the act of documenting our journey and honoring our victories serves as our compass and beacon. This chapter delves into the essence of progress tracking and the art of celebrating achievements, offering insights and practical strategies to enrich your expedition.

The Art of Progress Tracking: A Mirror to Our Journey

Documenting progress is akin to charting a map of our journey, providing clarity and direction. It's a reflective process that unveils the magnitude of our strides, the distance to our aspirations, and the adjustments required for our course. This practice is underpinned by research, such as a study in the Journal of Consulting and Clinical Psychology, highlighting that individuals who diligently monitored their progress were notably more successful in achieving their objectives compared to those who didn't.

Beyond goal attainment, progress tracking serves as a diagnostic tool, revealing patterns and habits that shape our journey. For instance, in the context of weight management, diligently logging dietary intake and physical activity sheds light on adherence to nutritional and fitness regimens, facilitating strategic tweaks to align with our goals.

The Joy of Celebrating Wins: Fueling Our Journey Forward

The act of celebrating achievements, irrespective of their magnitude, is a vital component of the journey. It's a ritual that acknowledges our dedication and progress, propelling us forward with renewed vigor. Small triumphs, be it surpassing a personal best in physical endeavors or reaching a new milestone in dietary discipline, deserve recognition. They serve as affirmations of our capabilities and fortify our resolve.

Moreover, the significance of celebrating wins transcends mere acknowledgement. Research published in the Journal of Personality and Social Psychology suggests that individuals who actively recognized and celebrated their progress were more likely to realize their ambitions swiftly, compared to those who overlooked their achievements.

- **Visual Progress Boards:** Create a visual representation of your progress and goals using a bulletin board or a digital app. Include photos, motivational quotes, and visual markers for each milestone you achieve. This serves as a daily visual reminder of where you've been and where you're headed.
- **Mindful Reflection Sessions:** Dedicate a weekly 15-minute session for mindful reflection on your progress. Use this time to meditate on your achievements, acknowledge the efforts you've put in, and set intentions for the coming week. This practice can deepen your connection to your journey and enhance your sense of fulfillment.
- **Personal Victory Dance:** Establish a personal "victory dance" or celebration ritual to perform every time you achieve a milestone, no matter how small. This physical expression of joy can boost your mood and make the act of achieving more memorable and fun.

- **Letter to Future Self:** Write letters to your future self at different stages of your journey, outlining your current achievements and hopes for the future. Open these letters upon reaching future milestones to reflect on your journey, recognize your growth, and motivate you to continue moving forward.
- **Create a 'Wins Jar':** Each time you achieve a goal, no matter how small, write it down on a piece of paper and place it in a 'Wins Jar.' Periodically, especially when in need of motivation, empty the jar and read through your wins. This tangible collection of achievements can serve as a powerful reminder of your progress and resilience.

By integrating these unique strategies into your journey, you not only track your progress and celebrate your achievements but also enrich your experience, making each step towards your goal a rewarding and enjoyable part of your personal growth narrative.

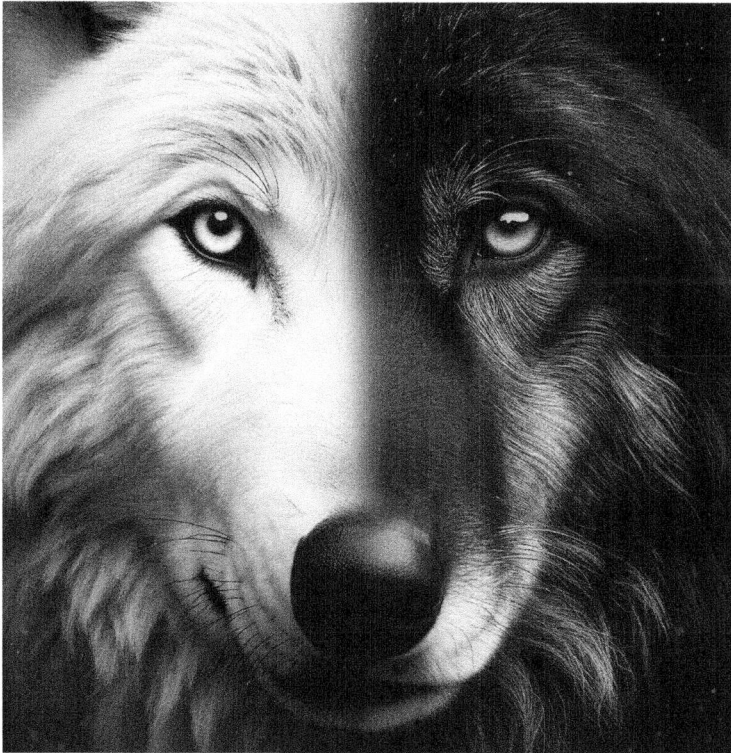

Daily Checklist (tick off)
☐ Meditation
☐ 10,000 Steps & Proof
☐ Wolf Workout
☐ Water Intake
☐ 8-Hour Eating Window
☐ Daily Learning (*Homework*)
☐ Supplements (*Optional*)
☐ 7+ Hours of Sleep
☐ Daily Progress Photo
☐ Alcohol & Sugar-Free

What visual symbol or item can you include on your Visual Progress Board this week to represent a recent achievement or milestone?

_____
_____
_____
_____
_____

Think of a moment from the past week you felt proud of. How can you incorporate this into your next Mindful Reflection Session?

_____
_____
_____
_____
_____

Reflecting on your progress so far, what specific win will you share with the Two Wolves Community today?

_____
_____
_____
_____

Journal the journey

Journal your thoughts on how you feel today and what steps you'll take to succeed tomorrow.

_____

_____

_____

_____

_____

_____

_____

_____

_____

_____

_____

_____

_____

_____

_____

_____

_____

_____

_____

_____

_____

_____

_____

_____

_____

_____

_____

_____

_____

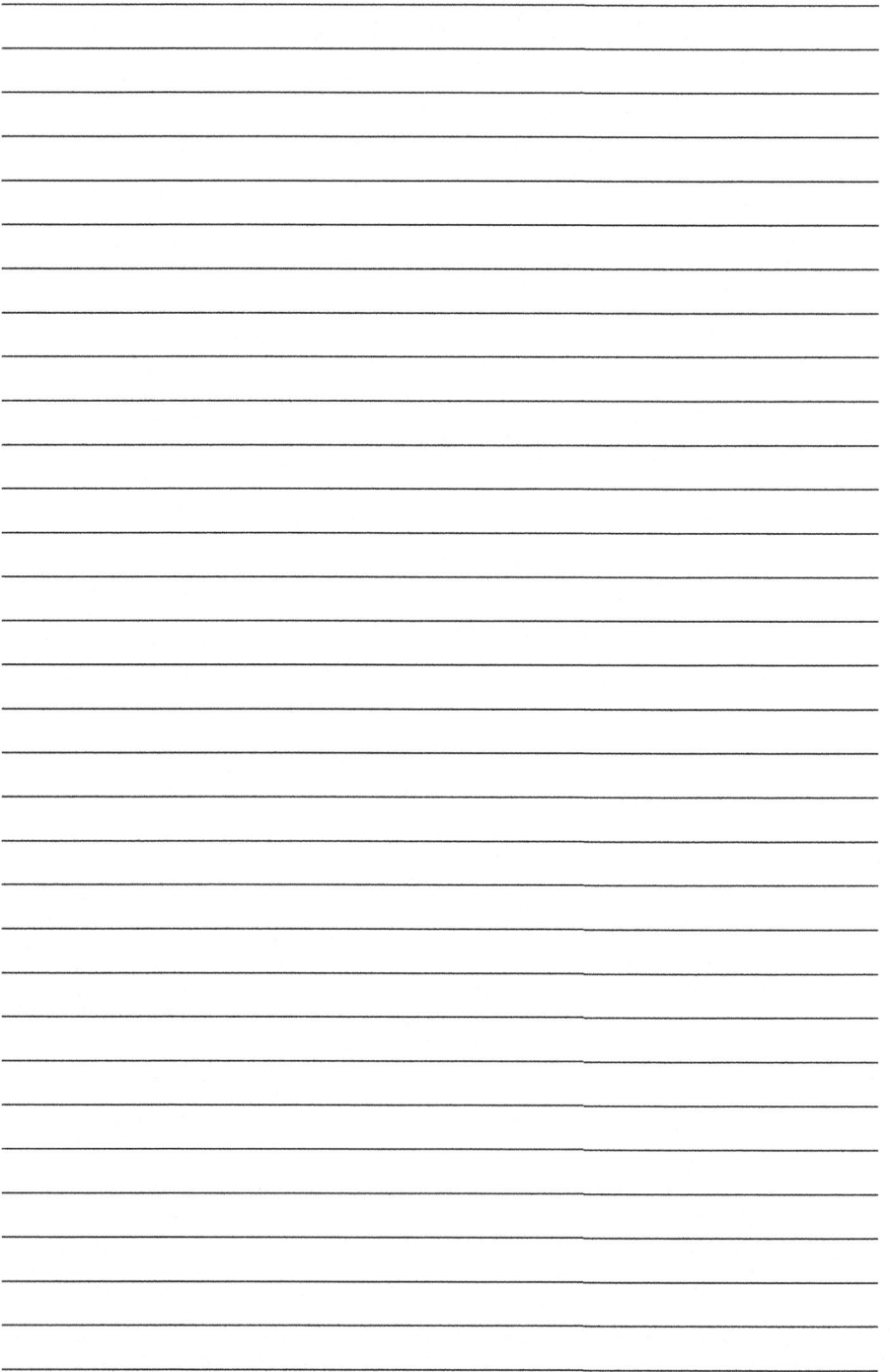

Day 14 Chapter 14
Wolf Unleashed

"The wolf on the hill is never as hungry as the wolf climbing the hill." - *Arnold Schwarzenegger*

Let's pause and reflect on the remarkable journey you've embarked upon. Beginning with a flicker of desire to transform, you've navigated through the wilderness of self-doubt, physical challenge, and mental fortitude. Approaching the midpoint is a testament to your perseverance and dedication.

The path has been anything but linear. With every stride, you've encountered a spectrum of emotions—pride in your achievements, trepidation for the road ahead, whispers of doubt questioning your capacity, and the physical and mental fatigue that accompanies any quest for change.

Embrace these feelings—they signify growth. You're undergoing a metamorphosis, shedding layers of your former self. It's in these moments of vulnerability that our true strength is forged. As Seneca the Younger once said, "It is not because things are difficult that we do not dare; it is because we do not dare that they are difficult." You dared to start this journey, proving your courage and resilience.

Amidst the ebb and flow of confidence, hold firm to the knowledge that retreat is not your destiny. You are not one to falter under adversity nor to accept anything less than what you've set out to achieve. You embody the spirit of the wolf—undaunted, steadfast, and relentless in pursuit of your goals.

As you move forward, reignite the spark that set you on this path. Recall the anticipation and the hunger for transformation that propelled you out of stasis. Marvel at your evolution, recognizing the strength you've cultivated and the barriers you've dismantled.

Celebrate yourself—every victory, every instance of personal growth, every obstacle overcome. These are the milestones of your journey, each one a testament to your indomitable will.

You are the embodiment of the unleashed wolf—majestic in your resolve, untamed in your ambition. Continue forth with unwavering determination. The horizon promises untold strength and fulfillment. The essence of your journey lies in the belief that "*The best way out is always through*" (Robert Frost).

Remember, you are not just journeying towards a destination but also cultivating the untapped potential within. You are the wolf unleashed—embrace your power.

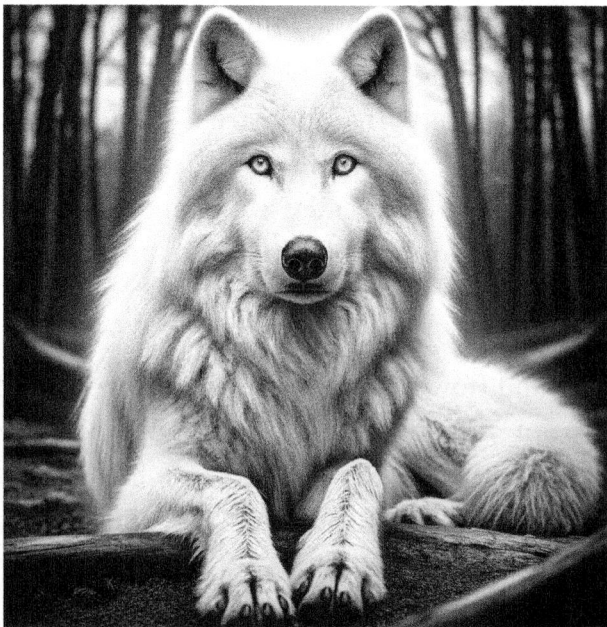

Daily Checklist (tick off)

☐ Meditation

☐ 10,000 Steps & Proof

☐ Wolf Workout

☐ Water Intake

☐ 8-Hour Eating Window

☐ Daily Learning (*Homework*)

☐ Supplements (*Optional*)

☐ 7+ Hours of Sleep

☐ Daily Progress Photo

☐ Alcohol & Sugar-Free

Reflecting on the past 14 days, what is one challenge you've overcome that you initially thought was insurmountable?

_____

_____

_____

_____

_____

How has your understanding of your personal strength and resilience evolved over the first half of this challenge?

._____

_____

_____

_____

Looking back at the progress you've made, what is one aspect of this journey that has surprised you the most about yourself?

_____

_____

_____

_____

Wolf Tracker 3

Congratulations on reaching this significant milestone in your Two Wolves journey! As you stand on the threshold of day 14, reflect on the strides you've made since you began. You've faced challenges head-on and shown remarkable dedication. Now, it's time to measure the progress you've made since day 1 and day 7, and set your sights on the path ahead with renewed determination and focus.

Date: _____

Push Ups
- Day 1: _____
- Day 7: _____
- Day 14: _____ (Record the number of push-ups you can perform in one minute.)

Squats
- Day 1: _____
- Day 7: _____
- Day 14: _____ (Record the number of squats you can perform in one minute.)

Jumping Jacks
- Day 1: _____
- Day 7: _____
- Day 14: _____ (Record the number of jumping jacks you can perform in one minute.)

Plank
- Day 1: _____
- Day 7: _____
- Day 14: _____ (Record the duration you can hold the plank position.)

Your journey through the Two Wolves program is a testament to your strength, resilience, and unwavering spirit. Each entry in this tracker is a step towards the best version of yourself.

Journal the journey

Journal your thoughts on how you feel today and what steps you'll take to succeed tomorrow.

_____
_____
_____
_____
_____
_____
_____
_____
_____
_____
_____
_____
_____
_____
_____
_____
_____
_____
_____
_____
_____
_____
_____
_____
_____
_____
_____
_____
_____
_____
_____
_____

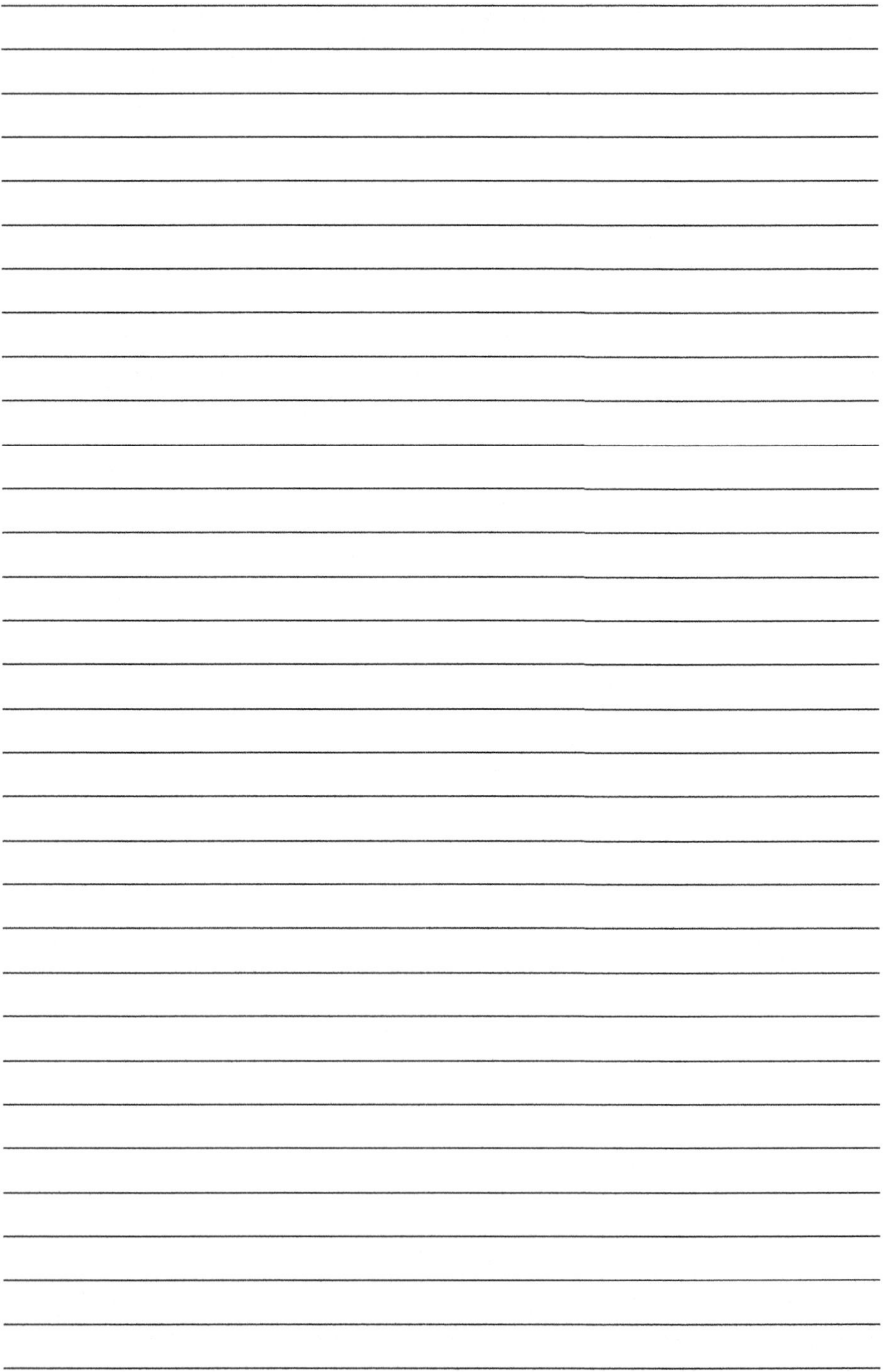

Wolf Workout Progression

Bravo on surmounting the challenges of Week 2 in your Wolf Workout journey! Each squat, push-up, leg raise, plank, and step-up brings you closer to embodying the strength and resilience of the wolf within. Now, it's time to elevate your training intensity as we move into Week 3, fostering greater growth, strength, and endurance.

Here's your updated **Wolf Workout regimen for Week 3**. This increment in reps and plank duration is meticulously planned to continue pushing your limits, ensuring ongoing progress without compromising your well-being.

- **Body Squats, Push-Ups, Leg Raises, and Step-Ups:** For these core exercises, you'll now be completing **5 sets of 7** repetitions each. This progression challenges your muscles further, enhancing strength, endurance, and muscle growth.
- **Elbow Plank:** This week, aim to hold the plank position for **40 seconds per set.** This increase fortifies core endurance and stability, laying a stronger foundation for all physical activities.

Week 3 beckons with new trials and triumphs. Remember, the journey of the wolf is not without its tests, but it is through these challenges that we find our true strength. Embrace this week's enhanced workout with the heart of a wolf—fierce, determined, and unwavering.

Your dedication to pushing past comfort zones and embracing growth mirrors the wolf's journey through uncharted forests. Keep the spirit of perseverance and resilience alive as you tackle Week 3, and let every rep remind you of the extraordinary capabilities within you.

Phase III

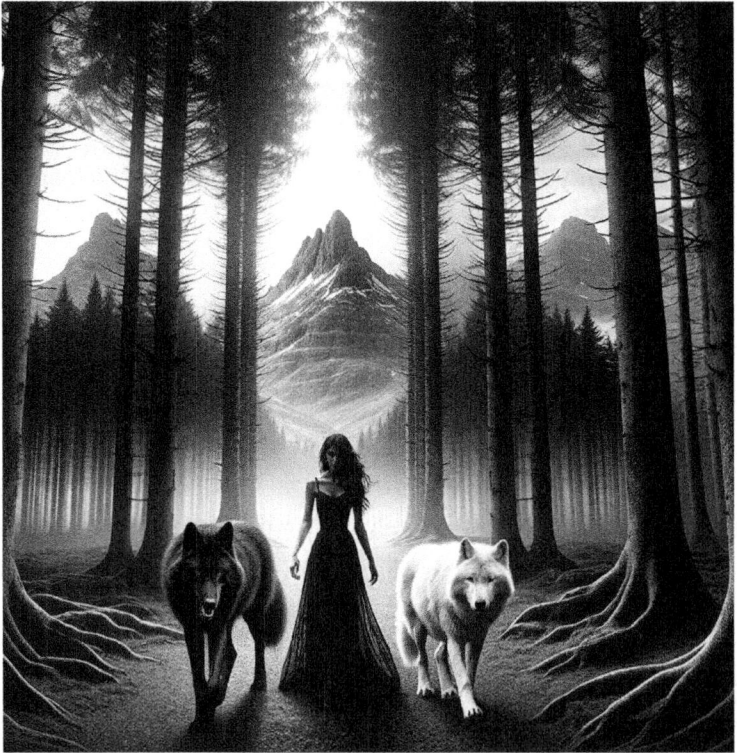

Empowerment

Day 15 Chapter 15
Overcoming Fear & Anxiety

"I learned that courage was not the absence of fear, but the triumph over it. The brave man is not he who does not feel afraid, but he who conquers that fear." -*Nelson Mandela*

In the labyrinth of human emotions, fear and anxiety often emerge as formidable foes, shaping our actions and influencing our decisions. Yet, within these feelings lies an opportunity for profound personal growth and transformation. Understanding fear and anxiety not as mere hindrances but as catalysts for change can fundamentally alter our journey towards self-realization and success.

The science of psychology provides a robust framework for understanding and navigating these complex emotions. Research suggests that fear, while uncomfortable, activates areas of the brain associated with decision-making and emotional regulation, such as the prefrontal cortex and amygdala. This activation is not meant to paralyze but to prepare us for action. Ancient wisdom aligns with this view, portraying fear as a test of courage and a step towards wisdom.

Exposure therapy, a concept with roots in both modern cognitive-behavioral therapy and timeless spiritual practices, exemplifies the proactive approach to fear. This method involves a gradual and repeated confrontation with the object of one's fear, in a controlled and supportive environment. Over time, this leads to a significant reduction in the emotional response to fear, illustrating the brain's remarkable capacity for neuroplasticity and adaptation.

Mindfulness meditation, deeply ingrained in ancient spiritual traditions and now embraced by contemporary science, offers a profound way to diminish the claws of anxiety and fear. Studies have shown that regular mindfulness practice can lead to structural changes in the brain, including increased density in areas related to attention, emotional regulation, and perspective-taking. This practice encourages a state of mindful observation, where fears are seen without judgment, reducing their intensity and impact.

Addressing the roots of fear and anxiety is pivotal. Often, our fears are tangled with internal narratives and past traumas that shape our perception of reality. Engaging with a mental health professional can unveil these underlying patterns, fostering a journey of healing and self-discovery. This therapeutic journey can be likened to the hero's quest, where confronting one's dragon leads to the treasure of deeper self-awareness and liberation.

Eleanor Roosevelt's immortal words, "*You gain strength, courage, and confidence by every experience in which you really stop to look fear in the face,*" echo through time, reminding us of the transformative power of confronting our fears. This confrontation is not a battle but a negotiation, leading to a greater understanding and mastery over our emotions.

Expanding Your Toolkit for Overcoming Fear and Anxiety:
- **Structured Exposure:** Incrementally increase your exposure to fears, documenting your feelings and reactions in a journal to track progress and insights.
- **Deepen Your Mindfulness Practice:** Engage in varied forms of mindfulness, including guided meditations, body scans, and mindful walking, exploring the nuances of your emotional landscape.

- **Cognitive Reframing:** Work with a therapist to identify and challenge limiting beliefs and cognitive distortions that fuel anxiety and fear.
- **Physiological Techniques:** Incorporate breathing exercises, yoga, or progressive muscle relaxation to reduce the physical manifestations of anxiety and fear.
- **Community Engagement:** Share your journey with a supportive community or group, fostering connections that provide empathy, understanding, and shared learning.

By delving deeper into the realm of fear and anxiety with intention and curiosity, we unlock the doors to our fullest potential. This journey is not one of eradication but of integration, embracing all facets of our being with compassion and courage. In doing so, we unleash our inner wolf – the embodiment of resilience, wisdom, and indomitable spirit – ready to lead us towards our destined path of fulfillment and triumph.

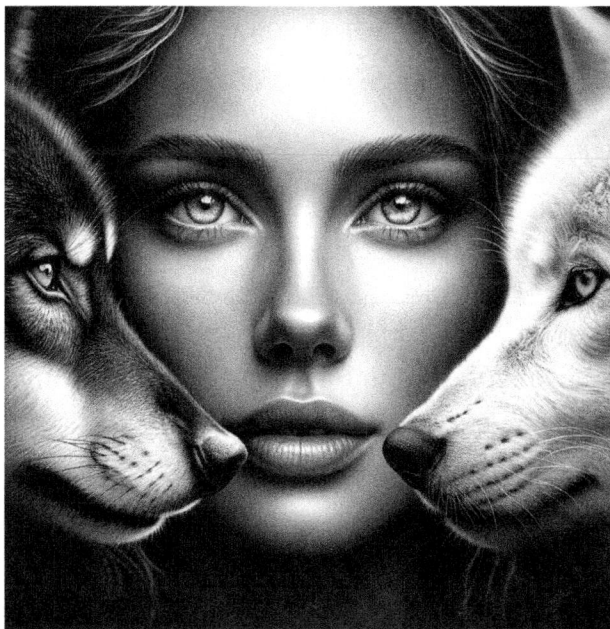

Daily Checklist (tick off)

☐ Meditation
☐ 10,000 Steps & Proof
☐ Wolf Workout
☐ Water Intake
☐ 8-Hour Eating Window
☐ Daily Learning (*Homework*)
☐ Supplements (*Optional*)
☐ 7+ Hours of Sleep
☐ Daily Progress Photo
☐ Alcohol & Sugar-Free

What specific fear will you commit to facing this week, and how will you gradually expose yourself to it?

_____

_____

_____

_____

_____

Reflect on a past experience where you overcame a fear. How did you feel afterward, and how can that success inspire your approach to current fears?.

_____

_____

_____

_____

_____

How are you feeling today, and what can you do to enhance your sense of well-being?

_____

_____

_____

_____

date ___ / ___ / ___

Journal the journey

Journal your thoughts on how you feel today and what steps you'll take to succeed tomorrow.

_____

_____

_____

_____

_____

_____

_____

_____

_____

_____

_____

_____

_____

_____

_____

_____

_____

_____

_____

_____

_____

_____

_____

_____

_____

_____

_____

_____

_____

_____

_____

_____

_____

_____

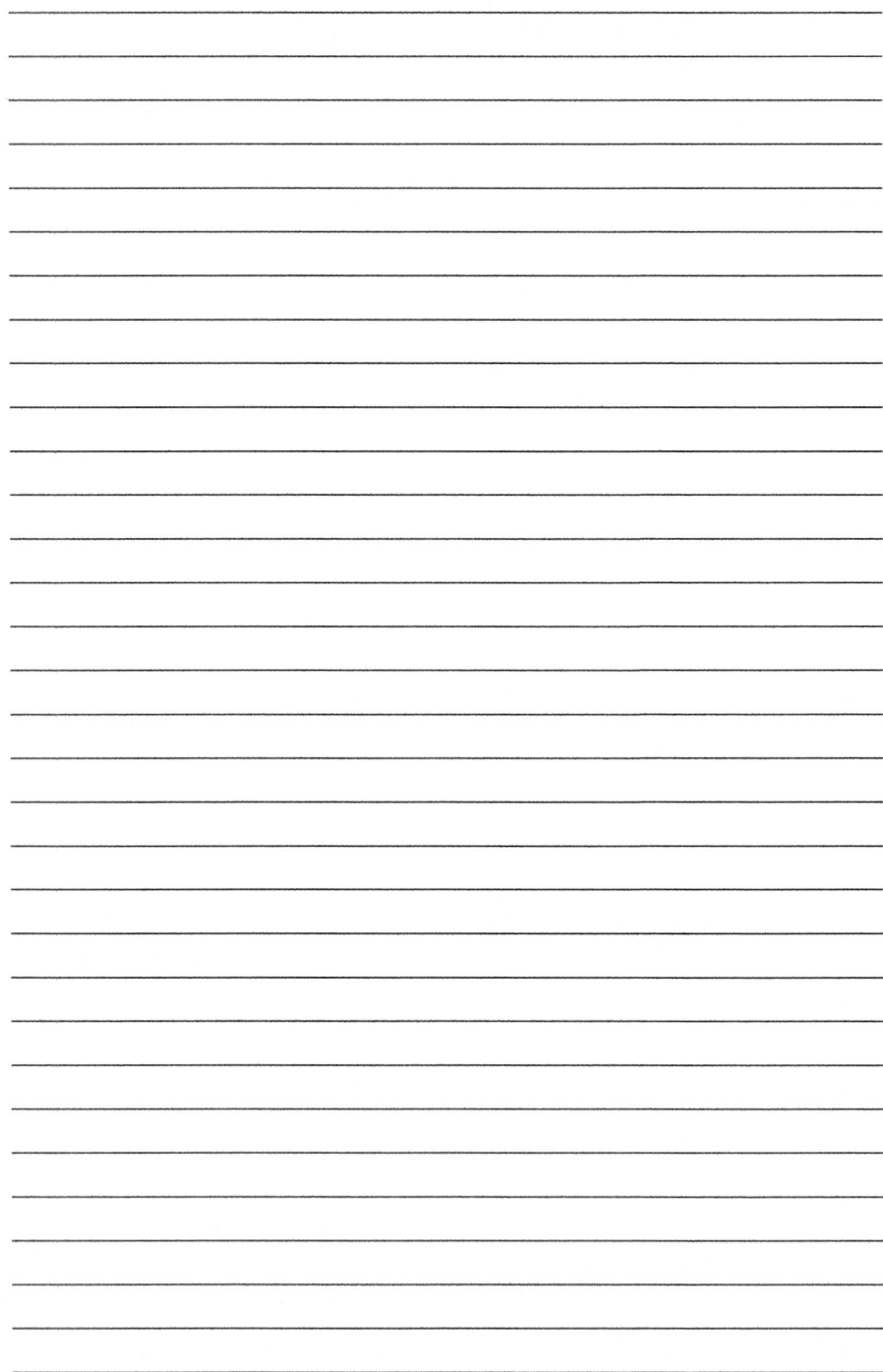

Day 16 Chapter 16
Quietening your inner critic
The Dark Wolf

"Your mind is a powerful thing. When you fill it with positive thoughts, your life will start to change." — *Gautama Buddha*

The narrative we hold within can either empower or constrain us, acting as a beacon of inspiration or a chain of self-doubt. This inner dialogue shapes our reality, guiding our actions and influencing our emotional state. The ancient wisdom of the Stoics, like Epictetus, reminds us, *"It's not what happens to you, but how you react to it that matters,"* underscoring the power of internal discourse over our external experiences. In modern times, neuroscience reveals that our self-talk can sculpt our brain's neural pathways, highlighting the tangible effects of our internal monologue on our mental and physical wellbeing.

Negativity within this internal dialogue can forge barriers to our happiness and success, tethering us to a cycle of self-criticism and diminished self-esteem. However, embracing strategies to cultivate a more supportive inner voice can liberate us from this cycle.

Practicing mindfulness, a technique with roots in ancient Buddhist traditions, enables us to witness our thoughts without attachment, granting us the clarity to discern between constructive self-reflection and detrimental self-judgment. Mindfulness allows us to exist in the moment, observing our inner critic as an outsider, and choosing not to engage with harmful narratives.

Engaging in cognitive restructuring, a concept widely supported by cognitive-behavioral therapy, encourages us to interrogate and reframe our negative thoughts. This process involves questioning the accuracy of our inner critic's admonishments and actively transforming these thoughts into affirmations of our capability and worth.

Cultivating self-compassion is paramount. Kristin Neff, a pioneering researcher on self-compassion, advocates treating ourselves with the same kindness and understanding during times of failure as we would a dear friend. This approach not only diminishes the power of the inner critic but also fosters resilience and a more positive self-view.

Creating a gratitude journal, as supported by numerous psychological studies, shifts focus from self-criticism to appreciation, enhancing our overall mental health and well-being. This practice encourages a habit of seeking out and acknowledging the positives in our life, thereby reducing the space available for the inner critic to thrive.

Lastly, seek feedback from trusted peers or mentors. This external perspective can provide a more balanced view of our actions and thoughts, offering reassurance and an alternative to the often distorted reflections of our inner critic.

In essence, the journey to silencing your inner critic is both an ancient quest and a modern challenge, bridging timeless wisdom with contemporary science. By harnessing mindfulness, challenging our negative thoughts, practicing self-compassion, fostering gratitude, and embracing external feedback, we can transform our inner dialogue into a source of strength and encouragement.

Remember, the power to change your narrative lies within you, echoing the timeless words of Mahatma Gandhi, *"Be the change that you wish to see in the world."* Let your inner voice be your guide, not your critic.

Actionable Tips:
- **Begin Each Day with Mindfulness:** Dedicate the first few minutes of your morning to mindfulness practice, setting a tone of awareness and presence for the day.
- **Challenge Negative Thoughts:** When a negative thought arises, pause and ask yourself, "Is this really true?" Challenge these thoughts and replace them with positive affirmations.
- **Practice Daily Self-Compassion:** Each evening, reflect on one act of kindness you showed yourself that day. This could be as simple as taking a break when needed or acknowledging your efforts.
- **Maintain a Gratitude Journal:** Write down three things you're grateful for each day. This practice can shift focus from criticism to appreciation.
- **Seek Constructive Feedback:** Regularly ask for feedback from people you trust. Use this as a learning tool to improve and balance your self-perception.

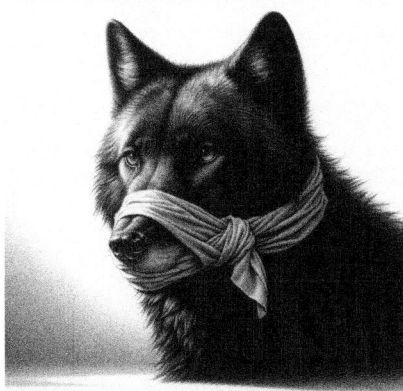

Daily Checklist (tick off)

☐ Meditation

☐ 10,000 Steps & Proof

☐ Wolf Workout

☐ Water Intake

☐ 8-Hour Eating Window

☐ Daily Learning (*Homework*)

☐ Supplements (*Optional*)

☐ 7+ Hours of Sleep

☐ Daily Progress Photo

☐ Alcohol & Sugar-Free

What specific thought patterns have you identified as the voice of your inner critic, and how do they impact your daily life?

_____

_____

_____

_____

_____

In what ways can you practice self-compassion today, especially after a setback or mistake?

_____

_____

_____

_____

_____

How has confronting your inner critic changed your approach to the challenges you've faced so far in this journey?

_____

_____

_____

_____

Journal the journey

Journal your thoughts on how you feel today and what steps you'll take to succeed tomorrow.

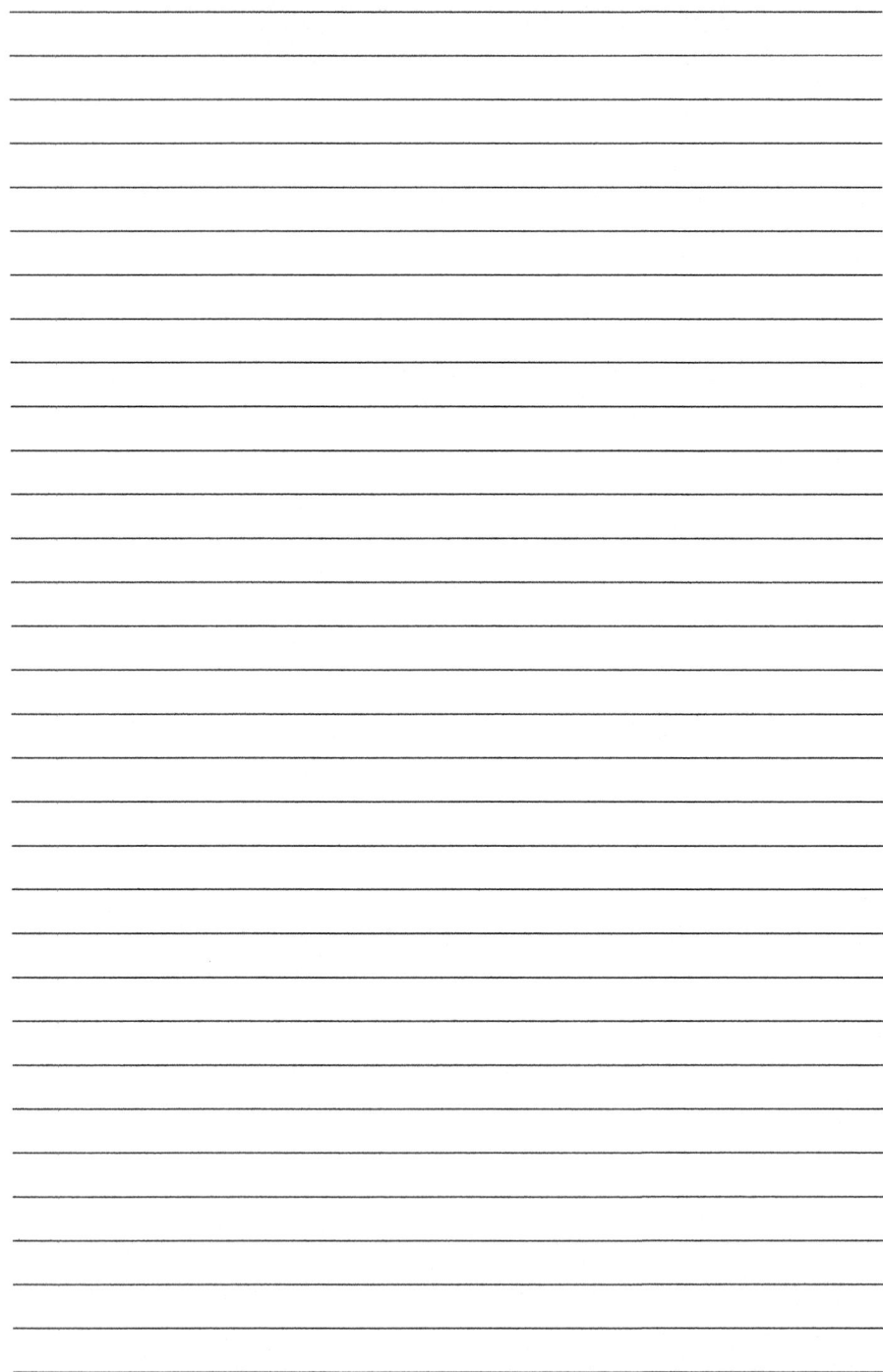

Day 17 Chapter 17
Developing Self-Compassion

"Love yourself first and everything else falls into line. You really have to love yourself to get anything done in this world."
— *Lucille Ball*

Developing self-compassion is akin to embarking on a transformative journey towards self-acceptance and inner peace. It is an ancient concept, endorsed by philosophers and sages from various traditions, and now robustly supported by a plethora of modern psychological research. The cultivation of self-compassion has been linked to numerous positive outcomes, including enhanced resilience, reduced psychological distress, and improved emotional well-being. Kristin Neff's pioneering work on self-compassion has emphasized its critical role in mental health, urging us to turn kindness inward.

Expand Mindfulness Practices: Beyond simple awareness, delve into practices that deepen mindfulness, such as guided meditations focusing specifically on self-compassion. The Buddhist tradition offers Metta (loving-kindness) meditation, which cultivates benevolence towards oneself and others. This practice has been scientifically shown to increase positive emotions and decrease negative ones.

Embrace Your Common Humanity: Recognize that imperfection and suffering are part of the shared human experience. Philosophers like Seneca and Epictetus emphasized the universality of human struggles, encouraging us to find strength in our shared vulnerabilities. Acknowledge that you are not alone in your feelings of inadequacy or failure; this realization fosters a more compassionate outlook towards yourself and others.

Cultivate a Forgiveness Practice: Integrating forgiveness into your self-compassion journey can have profound effects. Research in positive psychology highlights forgiveness as a pathway to releasing anger and resentment, including towards oneself. Practice forgiving yourself for past mistakes, and understanding that errors are opportunities for growth and learning.

Implement Compassion-focused Therapy (CFT) Exercises: Developed by Paul Gilbert, CFT is rooted in evolutionary psychology and neuroscience, offering specific exercises to cultivate warmth, safety, and a sense of soothing. These exercises, such as compassionate letter writing to oneself, encourage the development of a kinder, more understanding relationship with oneself.

Engage in Narrative Reconstruction: Inspired by the Stoic practice of journaling and modern narrative therapy, this involves writing about personal experiences with a focus on compassion and understanding. Reflect on past events and reframe them, emphasizing growth and forgiveness. This technique has been supported by research indicating that expressive writing can lead to improved mental health outcomes.

Create a Self-Compassion Ritual: Drawing on ancient ritualistic practices for inspiration, create a daily or weekly ritual focused on self-compassion. This could involve a quiet reflection on things you appreciate about yourself, a small ceremony of lighting a candle for self-acceptance, or a personal affirmation recited in front of a mirror.

Incorporating these practices into your life not only aligns with age-old wisdom but is also supported by contemporary scientific understanding. As Marcus Aurelius, the Stoic emperor, noted, "*Be tolerant with others and strict with yourself.*" This echoes the essence of self-compassion—holding space for our own imperfections while striving for personal growth and understanding. Through dedicated practice, we can navigate the path towards a more compassionate relationship with ourselves, grounded in both ancient wisdom and modern evidence.

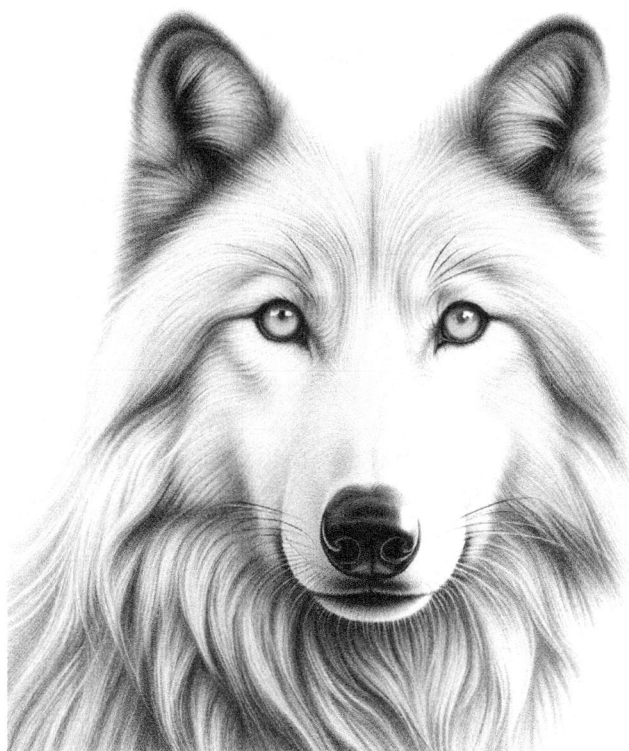

Daily Checklist (tick off)
☐ Meditation
☐ 10,000 Steps & Proof
☐ Wolf Workout
☐ Water Intake
☐ 8-Hour Eating Window
☐ Daily Learning (*Homework*)
☐ Supplements (*Optional*)
☐ 7+ Hours of Sleep
☐ Daily Progress Photo
☐ Alcohol & Sugar-Free

What is one kind thing you can say to yourself today?

_____

_____

_____

_____

_____

How can you incorporate self-compassion into your daily routine?

_____

_____

_____

_____

_____

What's one small step you can take to forgive yourself for a past mistake?

_____

_____

_____

_____

Journal the journey

Journal your thoughts on how you feel today and what steps you'll take to succeed tomorrow.

_____

_____

_____

_____

_____

_____

_____

_____

_____

_____

_____

_____

_____

_____

_____

_____

_____

_____

_____

_____

_____

_____

_____

_____

_____

_____

_____

_____

_____

_____

_____

_____

_____

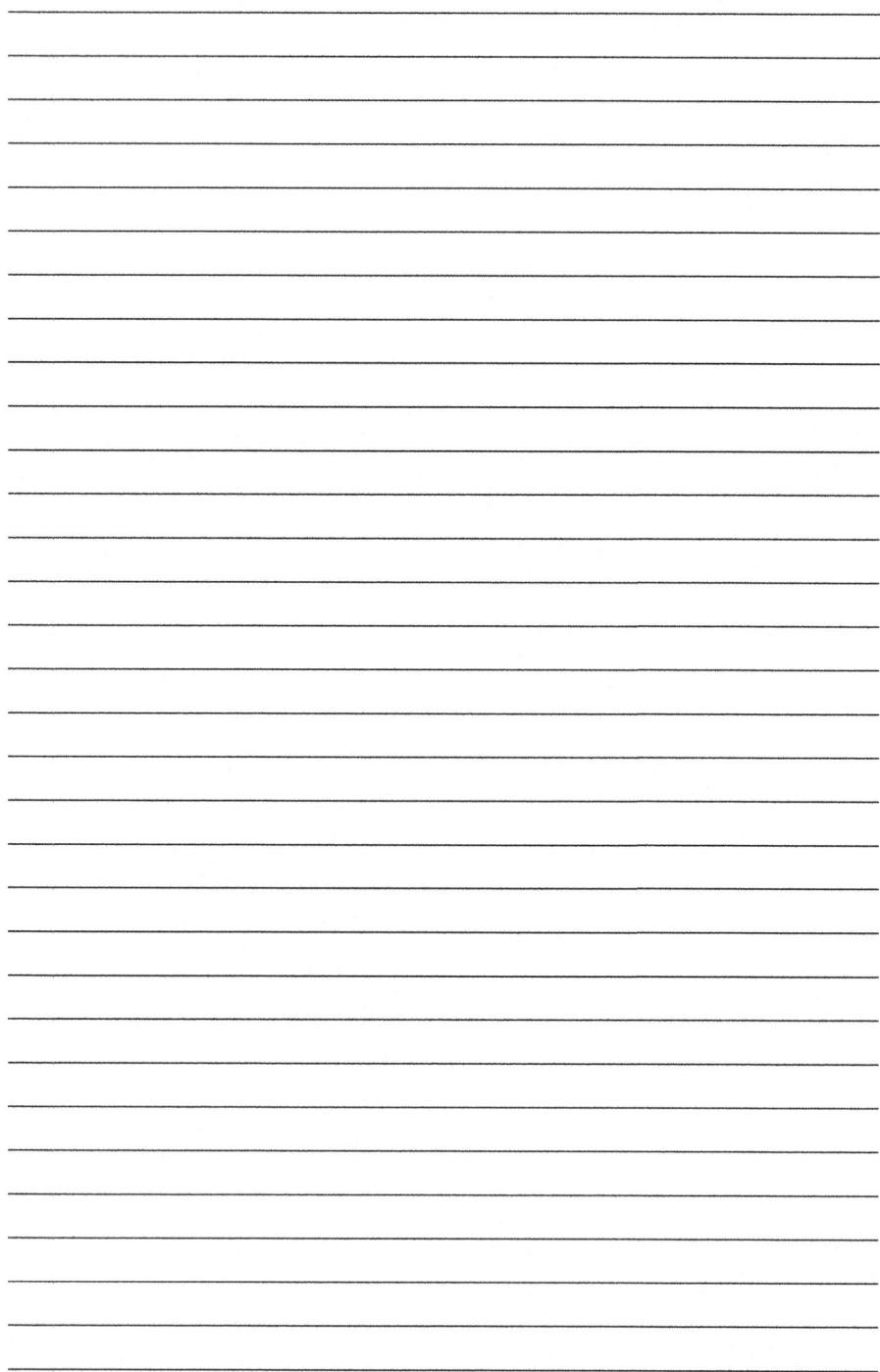

Day 18 Chapter 18 Choosing Light Over Darkness

"Out of suffering have emerged the strongest souls; the most massive characters are seared with scars." – *Khalil Gibran*

The battle between two primal forces within us—a luminescent wolf symbolizing virtues like courage and compassion, and its counterpart, a shadowy wolf fueling our fears and doubts—is a timeless allegory reflecting our internal struggles. This narrative not only highlights the dichotomy of human nature but also underlines the essence of resilience: the power to choose light over darkness, growth over stagnation.

Scientific research supports the notion that confronting rather than evading our internal battles fortifies mental resilience, enabling us to navigate life's adversities more effectively. A cornerstone study in Psychological Science illustrates that individuals who engage directly with their challenges exhibit higher levels of well-being and are more adept at managing stress compared to those who withdraw.

The concept of neuroplasticity, the brain's ability to reorganize itself by forming new neural connections throughout life, offers further insight into overcoming internal adversities. According to The Journal of Neuroscience, engaging in new, challenging activities stimulates neuroplasticity, reinforcing cognitive and emotional resilience. This scientific principle underscores the importance of confronting our shadow wolf, as each battle won strengthens our mental fortitude.

To integrate resilience into our lives and diminish the shadow wolf's influence, consider these scientifically backed strategies:

- **Structured Reflection:** Engage in daily reflective journaling, focusing on interactions with the shadow wolf. Neuroscience suggests that writing helps in emotional processing, allowing for a clearer understanding of our thoughts and behaviors (Harvard Medical School, 2018).
- **Embrace a Growth Mindset:** Adopting a growth mindset, the belief in our capacity to learn and grow from experiences, has been linked to greater resilience. Studies in Personality and Individual Differences show that individuals with a growth mindset are more persistent and less deterred by failure.
- **Forge Meaningful Connections:** The psychological theory of social support indicates that relationships play a pivotal role in resilience. A meta-analysis in Psychological Bulletin reveals that strong social connections are associated with reduced stress responses and increased emotional well-being.
- **Incorporate Mindfulness:** Mindfulness practices enhance emotional regulation and decrease reactivity to negative stimuli, as supported by research in Frontiers in Human Neuroscience. Regular mindfulness meditation can attenuate the influence of the shadow wolf by fostering a non-judgmental awareness of the present moment.
- **Acknowledge Progress:** Celebrating small victories is crucial in building resilience. According to The Journal of Positive Psychology, acknowledging personal growth moments enhances self-esteem and optimism, essential components in the resilience framework.

By employing these scientifically validated approaches, we not only counteract the shadow wolf's influence but also embark on a transformative journey towards a richer, more resilient existence. Embrace the words of Carl Jung, "*I am not what happened to me, I am what I choose to become,*" and let this wisdom guide you towards nurturing resilience and self-compassion. Through intentional action and reflection, we can harness the full spectrum of our inner strength, illuminating our path forward with the light wolf as our guide.

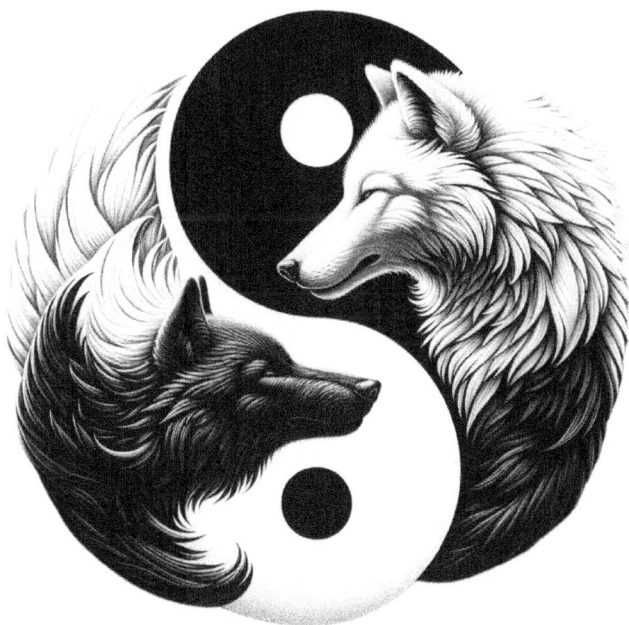

Daily Checklist (tick off)

☐ Meditation
☐ 10,000 Steps & Proof
☐ Wolf Workout
☐ Water Intake
☐ 8-Hour Eating Window
☐ Daily Learning (*Homework*)
☐ Supplements (*Optional*)
☐ 7+ Hours of Sleep
☐ Daily Progress Photo
☐ Alcohol & Sugar-Free

How do you currently cope with challenges? List one way you could improve this.

_____

_____

_____

_____

_____

What's one positive affirmation that resonates with you to counteract negative thoughts?"

_____

_____

_____

_____

_____

How are you feeling today, and how does that align with your goals for this challenge?

_____

_____

_____

_____

date ___ / ___ / ___

Journal the journey

Journal your thoughts on how you feel today and what steps you'll take to succeed tomorrow.

_____

_____

_____

_____

_____

_____

_____

_____

_____

_____

_____

_____

_____

_____

_____

_____

_____

_____

_____

_____

_____

_____

_____

_____

_____

_____

_____

_____

_____

_____

_____

_____

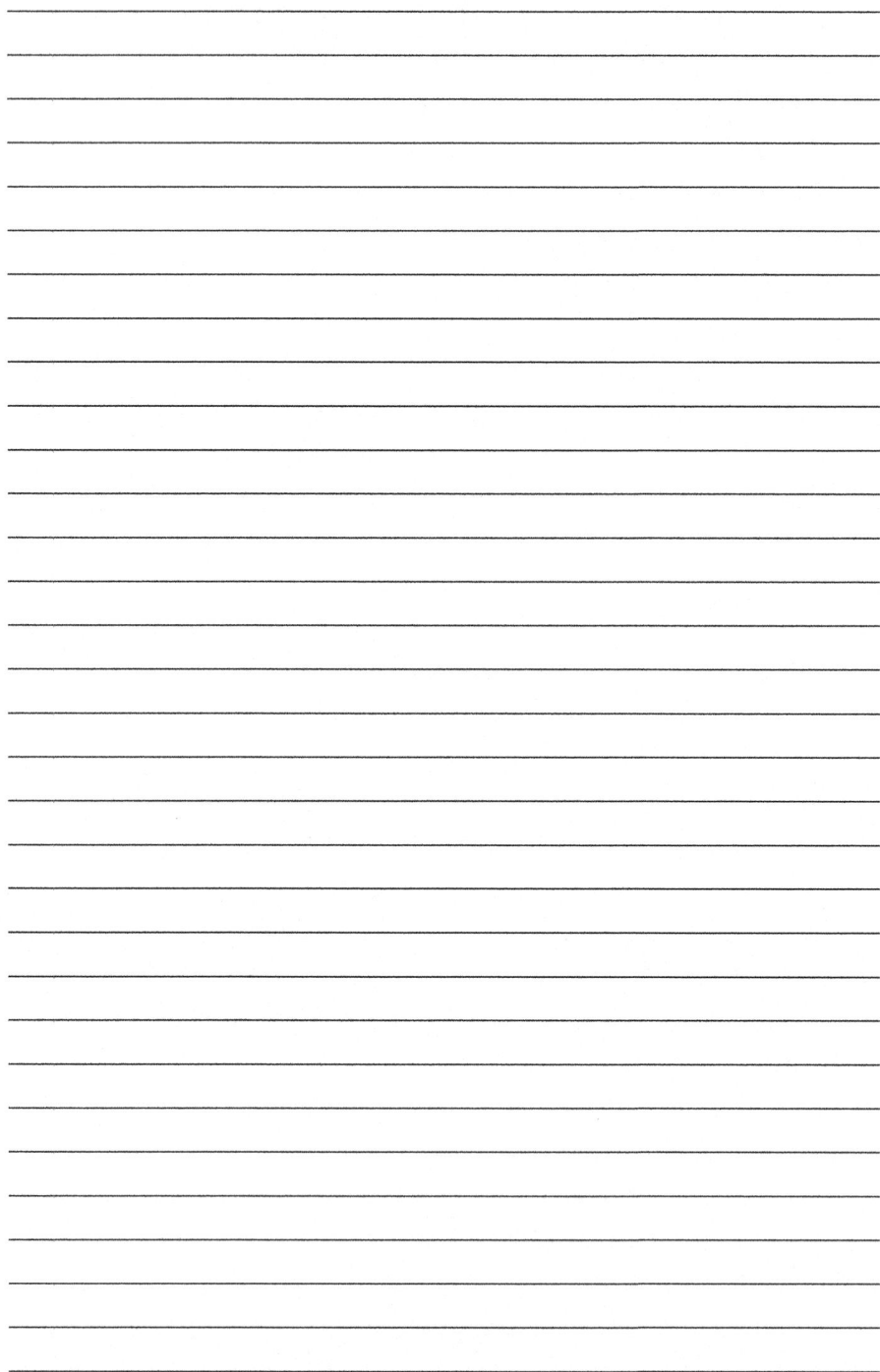

Day 19 Chapter 19
Mindful eating habits

"The food you eat can be either the safest and most powerful form of medicine or the slowest form of poison" - *Ann Wigmore*

Incorporating both ancient wisdom and cutting-edge scientific insights, our journey of mindful eating and intermittent fasting evolves into a profound exploration of our relationship with food and self. As we delve deeper into this chapter, we amplify our understanding and practice of these transformative habits, enhancing not only our physical health but our mental and spiritual well-being.

The Philosophical and Scientific Synergy of Mindful Eating and Intermittent Fasting

The 16/8 intermittent fasting method, where one consumes all daily calories within an eight-hour window followed by a sixteen-hour fast, is more than a dietary trend; it's a pathway to holistic health. This practice is underpinned by research from the Annual Review of Nutrition, which suggests that such fasting significantly improves metabolic health, aids in weight loss, and even contributes to longer lifespan by triggering cellular repair processes known as autophagy.

Meanwhile, mindful eating draws on ancient philosophies that view eating as a sacred act—a moment to connect with the essence of life. This approach to food consumption is about engaging all senses, acknowledging the journey of the food before it reaches the plate, and recognizing the nourishment it provides. A study in the Journal of Nutrition Education and Behavior found that individuals practicing mindful eating reported lower instances of emotional eating and made healthier food choices overall.

Deepening Practice: Integrating Mindful Eating with Intermittent Fasting

- **Begin with Intention:** Set a clear intention for your fasting and eating windows. Consider writing down what each meal represents to you beyond mere sustenance—perhaps a form of self-care, a moment of connection, or an act of gratitude toward the earth.

- **Holistic Nourishment Choices:** In your eating window, prioritize foods that not only nourish the body but also cater to the soul. Incorporate foods with a story—locally sourced produce, family recipes, or items that hold cultural significance, enhancing the mindfulness of your meals.

- **Cultivate Gratitude in Silence:** Dedicate the first few minutes of your eating window to silent reflection or a gratitude practice. Acknowledge the hands that cultivated your food, the elements that nurtured it, and the journey it undertook to become your nourishment.

- **Mindful Fasting Awareness:** During your fasting window, observe any arising thoughts or emotions related to food. Use this time for meditation or journaling to explore your relationship with hunger, satiety, and the emotional dimensions of eating.

- **Community Connection:** Share meals with loved ones or your pack when possible. Discuss the origins of your food, your reasons for intermittent fasting, and the insights you've gained through mindful eating. This communal practice can enrich the experience and foster a deeper connection to those around you.

As we navigate through the halfway mark of our transformative journey, the intertwining practices of mindful eating and intermittent fasting begin to manifest tangible results. Many report a renewed sense of energy, clarity of mind, and a deeper appreciation for the act of eating. It's crucial to celebrate these milestones, however small they may appear, as each step forward is a triumph over the past self—a gesture of commitment to growth and well-being.

Renowned mindfulness teacher Jon Kabat-Zinn eloquently captures the essence of this journey: *"Mindfulness means being awake. It means knowing what you are doing."* As we continue to awaken to the nuances of our eating habits and the rhythms of our bodies, we unleash a version of ourselves that is attuned not only to the needs of our physique but to the whispers of our spirit.

This chapter is not merely a set of instructions; it is an invitation to embark on a lifelong journey of discovery, where each meal becomes a reflection of our inner world and each moment of fasting a step toward self-realization. Embrace this path with an open heart, and let the ancient wisdom and scientific insights guide you toward a future where nourishment extends beyond the physical, touching the very core of your being.

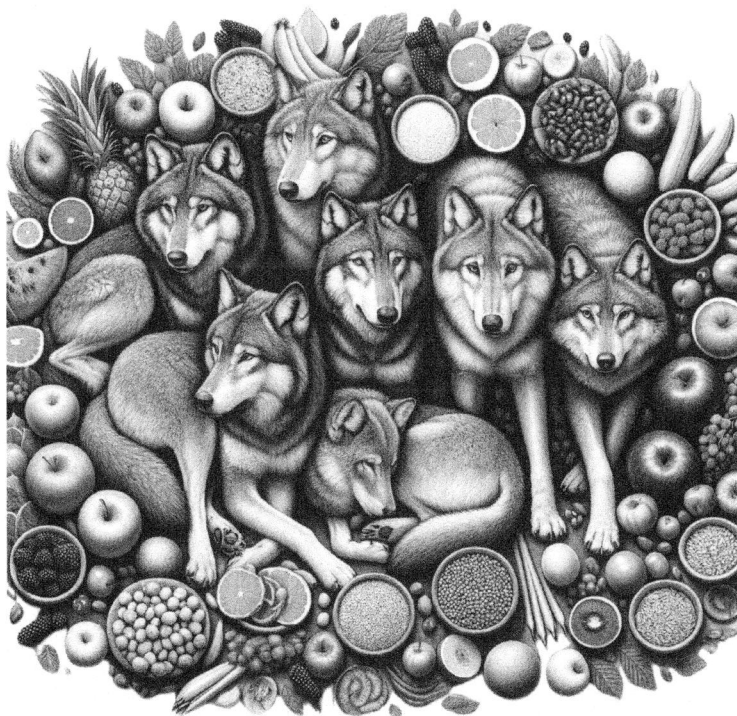

Daily Checklist (tick off)
☐ Meditation
☐ 10,000 Steps & Proof
☐ Wolf Workout
☐ Water Intake
☐ 8-Hour Eating Window
☐ Daily Learning (*Homework*)
☐ Supplements (*Optional*)
☐ 7+ Hours of Sleep
☐ Daily Progress Photo
☐ Alcohol & Sugar-Free

How has integrating mindful eating and intermittent fasting impacted your daily routine and overall sense of well-being?

_____

_____

_____

_____

_____

What changes have you noticed in your relationship with food since practicing these methods?

_____

_____

_____

_____

_____

In what ways can you further deepen your mindful eating practice during your next meal?

_____

_____

_____

_____

Journal the journey

Journal your thoughts on how you feel today and what steps you'll take to succeed tomorrow.

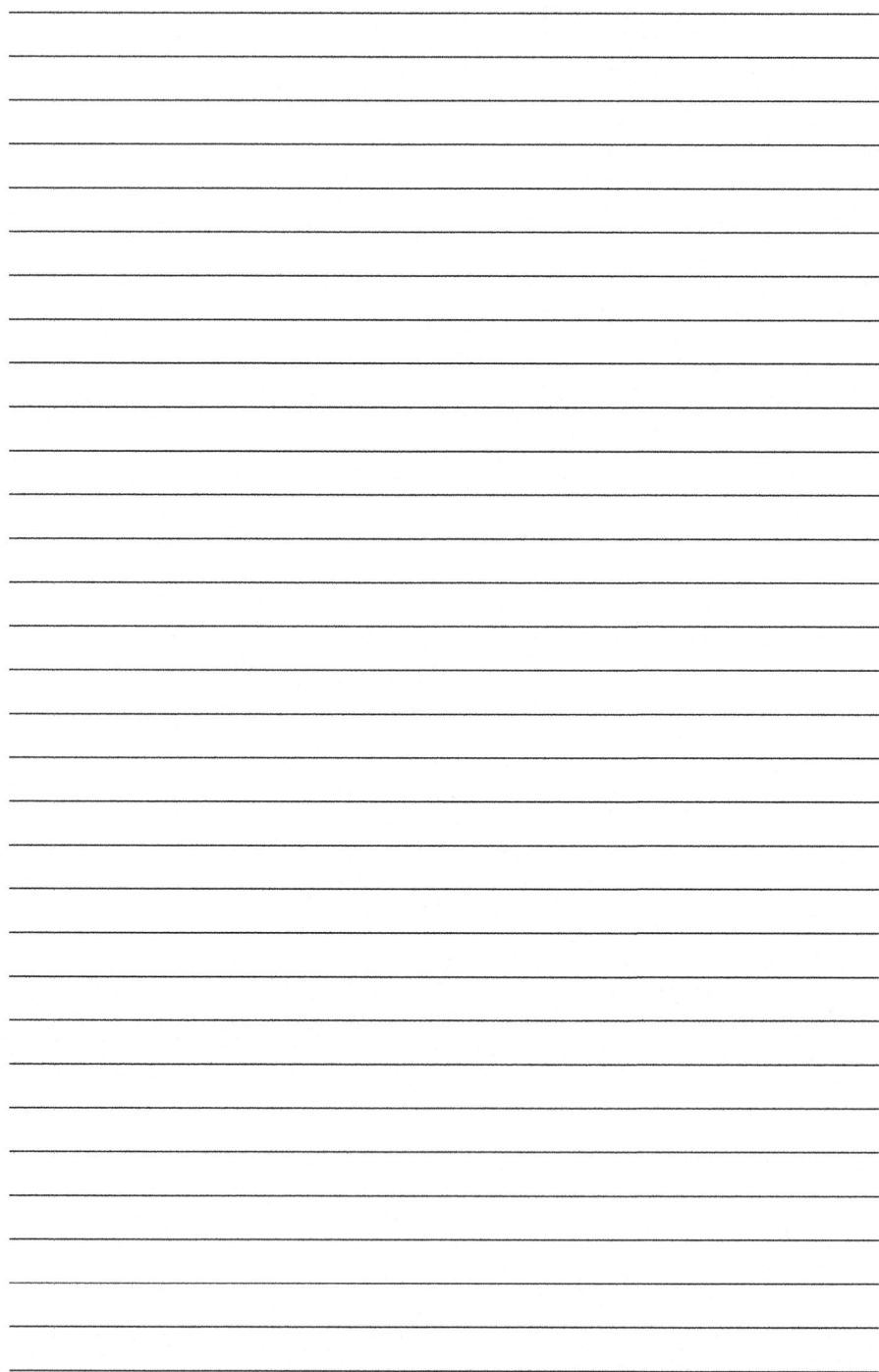

Day 20 Chapter 20
Managing Stress

"Rule number one is, don't sweat the small stuff. Rule number two is, it's all small stuff." - *Robert Eliot*

Stress, the shadowy figure that walks alongside every human endeavor, can be a formidable foe. Its presence is as ancient as humanity itself, yet our understanding and strategies to manage it have evolved significantly. Ancient wisdom teaches us that life's challenges are not to be avoided but embraced as pathways to growth. Modern science backs this up, showing us concrete ways to mitigate stress and turn it into a catalyst for resilience and achievement.

Mindfulness Meditation: The Anchor in Stormy Seas Mindfulness meditation is not just a practice but a refuge. The Journal of Psychosomatic Medicine has documented its efficacy in reducing stress markers in the body. By anchoring your awareness in the present, you can observe life's tumult without being swept away, transforming reactive patterns into thoughtful responses.

Exercise: The Alchemy of Stress into Strength Exercise is the alchemist that turns the leaden weight of stress into the gold of vitality. The Harvard Medical School highlights its dual role in reducing the physical symptoms of stress and elevating mood through the release of endorphins. Whether it's a brisk walk or a vigorous workout, movement is a powerful spell to dispel the clouds of stress.

Deep Breathing: The Calm Within the Storm Deep breathing is a simple yet profound technique to navigate stress.

The American Institute of Stress points out its capacity to lower cortisol levels, inviting calm and focus. In moments of tension, deep, rhythmic breaths can be a lifeline back to tranquility.

Progressive Muscle Relaxation: Easing the Tides of Tension Progressive muscle relaxation is a technique recommended by the Mayo Clinic for its effectiveness in reducing stress-induced muscle tension. By methodically tensing and relaxing muscle groups, you can release stress physically and mentally, reminding your body of its natural state of relaxation.

Aromatherapy: Scents of Serenity Aromatherapy offers a gentle yet powerful way to soothe the mind. Research published in the Journal of the International Society of Sports Nutrition highlights lavender's role in reducing stress and promoting sleep. Scent can be a direct pathway to calm, offering immediate relief with just a few deep breaths.

Implementing these techniques into your daily life can transform the way you experience and manage stress. They serve not just as tools but as stepping stones to a more balanced, resilient life. Embrace these practices with the heart of an explorer, and let the journey toward mastering stress begin.

Actionable Tips:
- **Start Small:** Begin with your mindfulness meditation each day, gradually increasing the time as you feel more comfortable.
- **Integrate Movement:** Incorporate short, daily walks or a preferred form of exercise into your routine to engage body and mind.
- **Breathe with Purpose:** Practice deep breathing techniques during moments of high stress to instantly lower your stress levels.

- **Schedule Relaxation:** Make progressive muscle relaxation a regular part of your evening routine to ensure restful sleep.
- **Create a Sanctuary:** Use aromatherapy in your living space to create a calming environment that counteracts stress.

"Stress is not a state of the world but a state of mind. We control it, not by changing the world, but by managing our thoughts." - Adapted from an ancient proverb, this reminder serves as a beacon of wisdom, guiding us to find peace amidst chaos.

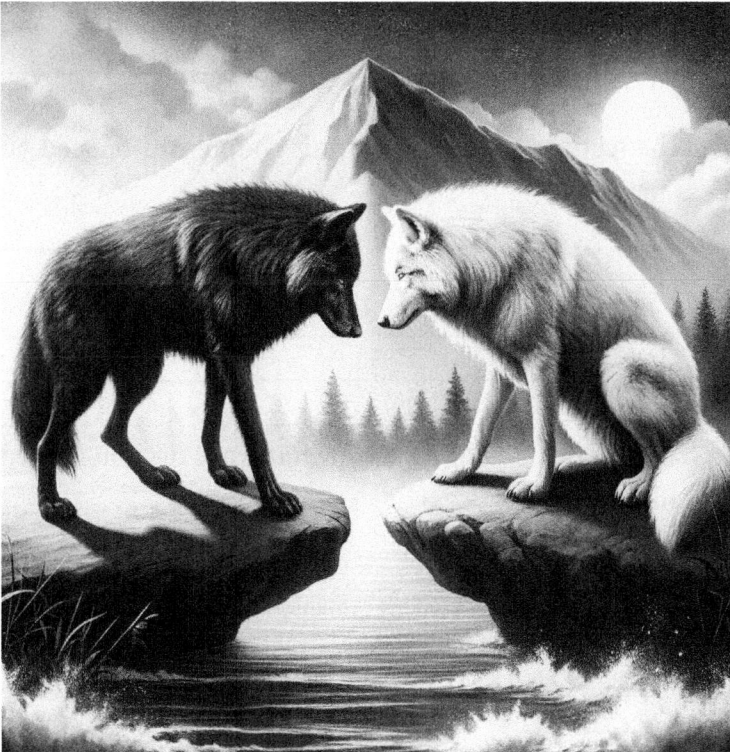

Daily Checklist (tick off)
- ☐ Meditation
- ☐ 10,000 Steps & Proof
- ☐ Wolf Workout
- ☐ Water Intake
- ☐ 8-Hour Eating Window
- ☐ Daily Learning (*Homework*)
- ☐ Supplements (*Optional*)
- ☐ 7+ Hours of Sleep
- ☐ Daily Progress Photo
- ☐ Alcohol & Sugar-Free

What has been the most stress-inducing aspect of this program for you so far? How did you manage it?

_____

_____

_____

_____

_____

How have the techniques learned in this chapter influenced your daily stress levels?

_____

_____

_____

_____

Looking back on the last 20 days, in what ways do you feel you've grown or changed?

_____

_____

_____

_____

Journal the journey

Journal your thoughts on how you feel today and what steps you'll take to succeed tomorrow.

_____

_____

_____

_____

_____

_____

_____

_____

_____

_____

_____

_____

_____

_____

_____

_____

_____

_____

_____

_____

_____

_____

_____

_____

_____

_____

_____

_____

_____

_____

_____

_____

_____

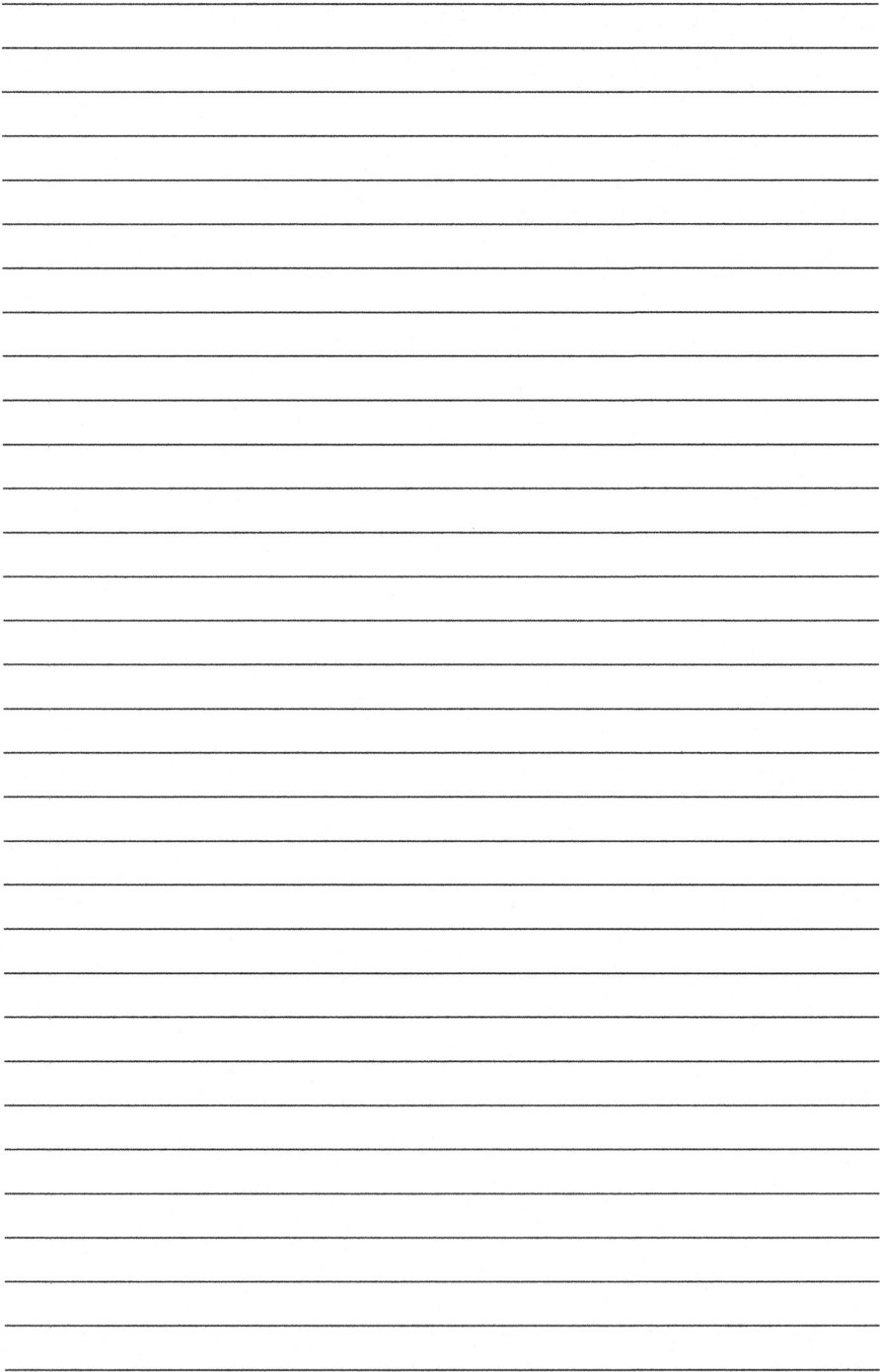

Day 21 Chapter 21
Habits Formed

"The only person you are destined to become is the person you decide to be." – *Ralph Waldo Emerson*

Congratulations on reaching Day 21 of your journey. Today marks a significant milestone, not just in this challenge, but in the landscape of your personal growth. According to popular belief, backed by some psychological research, it takes about 21 days to form a new habit. While the science of habit formation is complex and varies from person to person, the 21-day mark is a powerful symbol of transformation and renewal. You've been feeding the good wolf consistently, and now, you're beginning to see the fruits of your labor.

The genesis of the 21-day concept traces back to Dr. Maxwell Maltz's observations in the 1960s, as outlined in his book "Psycho-Cybernetics." Dr. Maltz noticed that patients took approximately 21 days to adjust to a new physical change. Although more recent research suggests that the time it takes to form a habit can vary widely, the 21-day mark has become a motivational milestone, encouraging individuals to persist in their efforts to make positive changes.

Now, as you stand at this pivotal point, it's time to reflect on the journey that has led you here and to look forward to the path that lies ahead. Every moment is an opportunity to be a new you, to choose which wolf to feed, and to live in alignment with your deepest values and aspirations.

Science of New Habits

The process of habit formation is grounded in the science of neuroplasticity, the brain's ability to reorganize itself by forming new neural connections throughout life. Repetitive behavior strengthens these connections, gradually making new behaviors automatic. This transformation is at the heart of what it means to cultivate new habits and shed old ones that no longer serve us.

Embracing the New You

With each day, you've been writing a new chapter in the story of your life, choosing actions that align with your aspirations and values. The new you is not a distant dream but a present reality, continually evolving with every choice you make. Embrace this process of becoming, knowing that each step forward is a step into the person you are meant to be.

Making It Fun and Inspirational

- **Celebrate Your Progress:** Take time to celebrate your achievements, no matter how small. Celebrating reinforces positive behavior and keeps you motivated.
- **Share Your Journey:** Sharing your progress with the Two Wolves community can inspire others and provide you with support and encouragement. Your story is powerful.
- **Visualize Your Success:** Spend a few minutes each day visualizing your success. Imagining your goals as already achieved can boost your motivation and help solidify your commitment to your new habits.
- **Be Kind to Yourself:** Practice self-compassion. If you stumble, treat yourself with the same kindness you would offer a friend. Each day is a new opportunity to continue your journey.
- **Keep Exploring:** Stay curious and open to trying new techniques, activities, or routines that can enrich your journey. Life is an adventure; embrace the learning that comes with it.

As you move forward, remember that every day is an opportunity to feed the good wolf, to make choices that align with your highest self, and to embrace the endless process of becoming. You are a testament to the power of persistence, the beauty of transformation, and the strength of the human spirit. Here's to you, the new you, on Day 21 and beyond. Awoo!

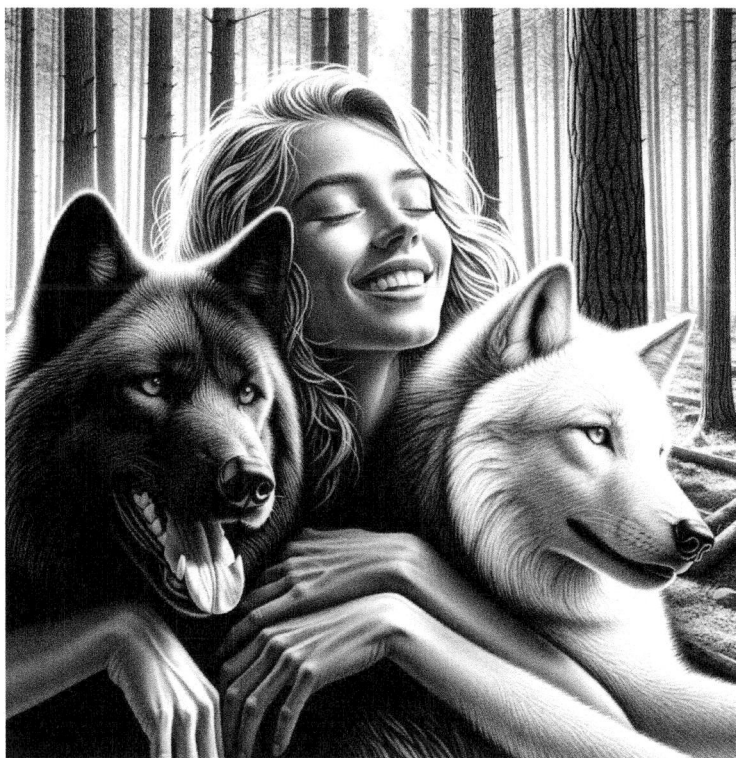

Daily Checklist (tick off)

☐ Meditation

☐ 10,000 Steps & Proof

☐ Wolf Workout

☐ Water Intake

☐ 8-Hour Eating Window

☐ Daily Learning (*Homework*)

☐ Supplements (*Optional*)

☐ 7+ Hours of Sleep

☐ Daily Progress Photo

☐ Alcohol & Sugar-Free

Reflecting on the past 21 days, what new habit are you most proud of developing, and how has it impacted your daily life?

_____

_____

_____

_____

_____

How have the changes you've implemented over the last three weeks altered your perspective on health, wellness, and personal growth?

_____

_____

_____

_____

_____

What was the most challenging habit to incorporate into your routine, and how did you overcome the obstacles to make it a consistent part of your life?

_____

_____

_____

_____

Wolf Tracker 4

Congratulations on reaching this pivotal point in your Two Wolves journey! Day 21 marks a transformative phase where the habits you've been nurturing have begun to solidify, shaping you into a newer version of yourself.

Date: _____

Push Ups Day 1: _____

Day 7: _____

Day 14: _____

Day 21: _____ (Record the number of push-ups you can perform in one minute.)

Squats

Day 1: _____

Day 7: _____

Day 14: _____

Day 21: _____ (Record the number of squats you can perform in one minute.)

Jumping Jacks

Day 1: _____

Day 7: _____

Day 14: _____

Day 21: _____ (Record the number of jumping jacks you can perform in one minute.)

Plank Day 1: _____

Day 7: _____

Day 14: _____

Day 21: _____ (Record the duration you can hold the plank position.)

Keep pushing, keep growing, and remember—the best is yet to come. We are nearly at the peak of this challenge, let's go wolf cub! Let's Go! Awooooo!

Journal the journey

Journal your thoughts on how you feel today and what steps you'll take to succeed tomorrow.

_____
_____
_____
_____
_____
_____
_____
_____
_____
_____
_____
_____
_____
_____
_____
_____
_____
_____
_____
_____
_____
_____
_____
_____
_____
_____
_____
_____
_____
_____

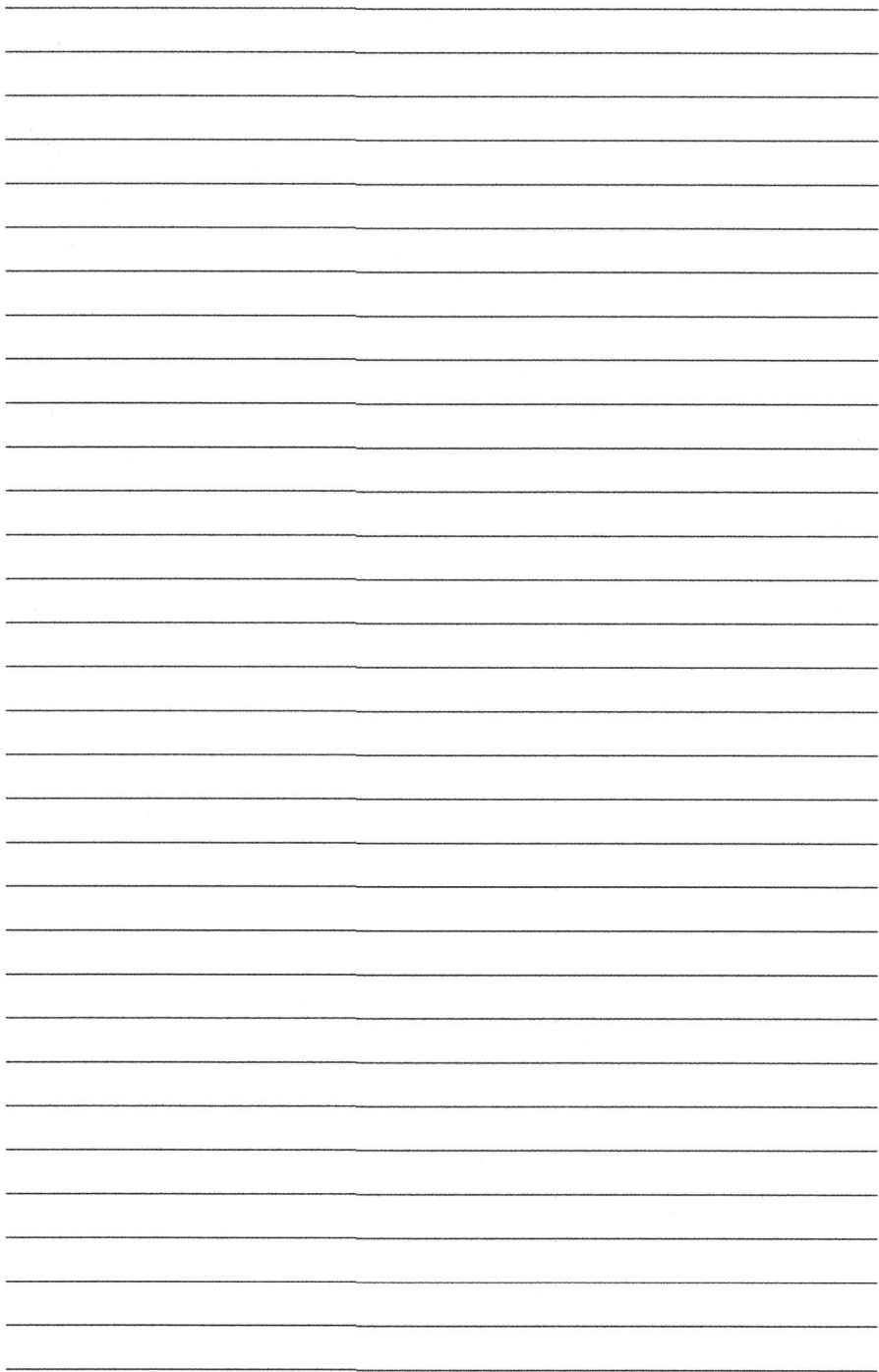

Wolf Workout Progression

Congratulations on reaching the final stretch of your Wolf Workout progression! Your journey thus far is a testament to your determination, growth, and the relentless spirit of the wolf. As you gear up for Week 4, let's elevate the intensity one last time, pushing through to the pinnacle of your current capabilities.

Here's your challenge for Week 4, designed to solidify the gains you've made and test the boundaries of your endurance and strength.

- **Body Squats, Push-Ups, Leg Raises, and Step Ups:** This week, you're tasked with completing **5 sets of 8 repetitions** for each of these exercises. This final increase is aimed at maximizing muscle endurance, strength, and overall physical fitness.

- **Elbow Plank:** Your goal is to hold the plank position for a challenging **45 seconds per set**. This significant jump in duration is crucial for enhancing core strength, improving posture, and stabilizing your entire body.

As you embark on this final week of intensified training, remember the essence of the wolf spirit—its resilience, its endurance, and its ability to lead and thrive. Let these qualities inspire you to embrace each day's workout with enthusiasm and resolve.

This week is not just a culmination of your efforts but a gateway to new beginnings and further achievements. The discipline, strength, and resilience you've built are qualities that will serve you well beyond this program.

Embrace this final week with the courage and tenacity of a wolf facing the dawn. You are not at the end of a journey, but at the beginning of a lifelong path of strength, health, and relentless pursuit of your best self. Awoo!

Phase IV

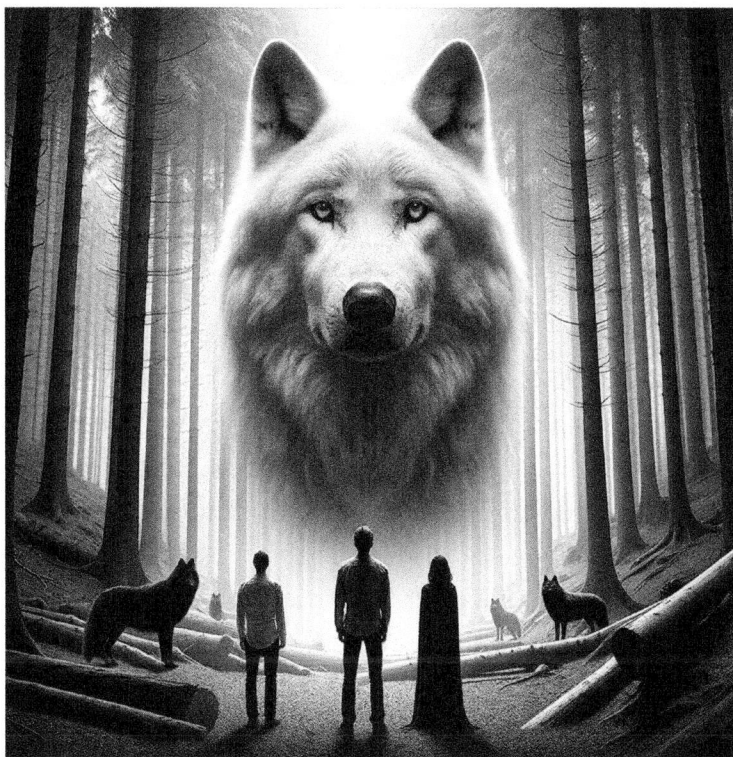

Mastery

Day 22 Chapter 22
Advancing Your Level

"Strength does not come from physical capacity. It comes from an indomitable will." – *Mahatma Gandhi*

As we embark on the final stretch of this transformative journey, the ancient wisdom, "*The journey of a thousand miles begins with a single step,*" resonates deeply. You've already taken numerous steps on this path, and now, it's time to intensify your efforts, refine your focus, and truly step up your game. The final phase is not just another segment of your journey; it's the pinnacle of your dedication, where every bit of hard work converges to catapult you toward your ultimate fitness goals.

Sharpen Your Focus: Now, more than ever, it's critical to hone your focus. Distractions are the adversaries of progress. Remind yourself of your goals daily, visualize your success, and reaffirm your commitment to achieving them. This is your moment to shine.

Enhance Nutritional Vigilance: Nutrition plays a pivotal role in your ability to perform and recover. As you push your limits, your body demands more. Optimize your nutrition to fuel your intensified workouts. Remember the adage, "You can't out-train a bad diet." Nourish your body with precision.

Refine and Intensify Workouts: Elevate the intensity of your workouts. If you've been comfortably meeting your workout targets, it's time to push beyond. Increase the reps, extend the planks, and incorporate more challenging exercises. Embrace the discomfort; it's a harbinger of progress.

Cultivate Resilience and Grit: Resilience and grit are your allies in this final push. Challenges will arise, but your response to these hurdles defines your journey. As Winston Churchill wisely stated, *"Success is not final, failure is not fatal: It is the courage to continue that counts."*

Seek Joy in the Journey: Find joy in the rigor and the challenge. The satisfaction of pushing past what you once thought impossible is unparalleled. Let this joy fuel your final stretch.

This is the crescendo of your fitness symphony, a time to amplify your efforts and truly transcend your previous limitations. Let the words of Nelson Mandela inspire you: *"It always seems impossible until it's done."* You're on the cusp of transforming the impossible into your new reality.

Remember, this final stretch is not just about reaching the finish line; it's about how much you can push yourself to achieve heights of fitness and well-being you've never experienced before. Every day, every workout, every mindful meal is an opportunity to excel. Feed your good wolf, embrace the challenge, and unleash the fullest potential of your inner strength. The best is yet to come.

Daily Checklist (tick off)

☐ Meditation
☐ 10,000 Steps & Proof
☐ Wolf Workout
☐ Water Intake
☐ 8-Hour Eating Window
☐ Daily Learning (*Homework*)
☐ Supplements (*Optional*)
☐ 7+ Hours of Sleep
☐ Daily Progress Photo
☐ Alcohol & Sugar-Free

Reflect on a moment during this challenge when you felt you surpassed your limits. How can you use that experience to drive you in this final stretch?

_____

_____

_____

_____

_____

How can you adjust your nutrition plan this week to better fuel your intensified workouts?

_____

_____

_____

_____

How are you feeling about your progress as we enter the final stretch of the challenge?

_____

_____

_____

_____

Journal the journey

Journal your thoughts on how you feel today and what steps you'll take to succeed tomorrow.

_____

_____

_____

_____

_____

_____

_____

_____

_____

_____

_____

_____

_____

_____

_____

_____

_____

_____

_____

_____

_____

_____

_____

_____

_____

_____

_____

_____

_____

_____

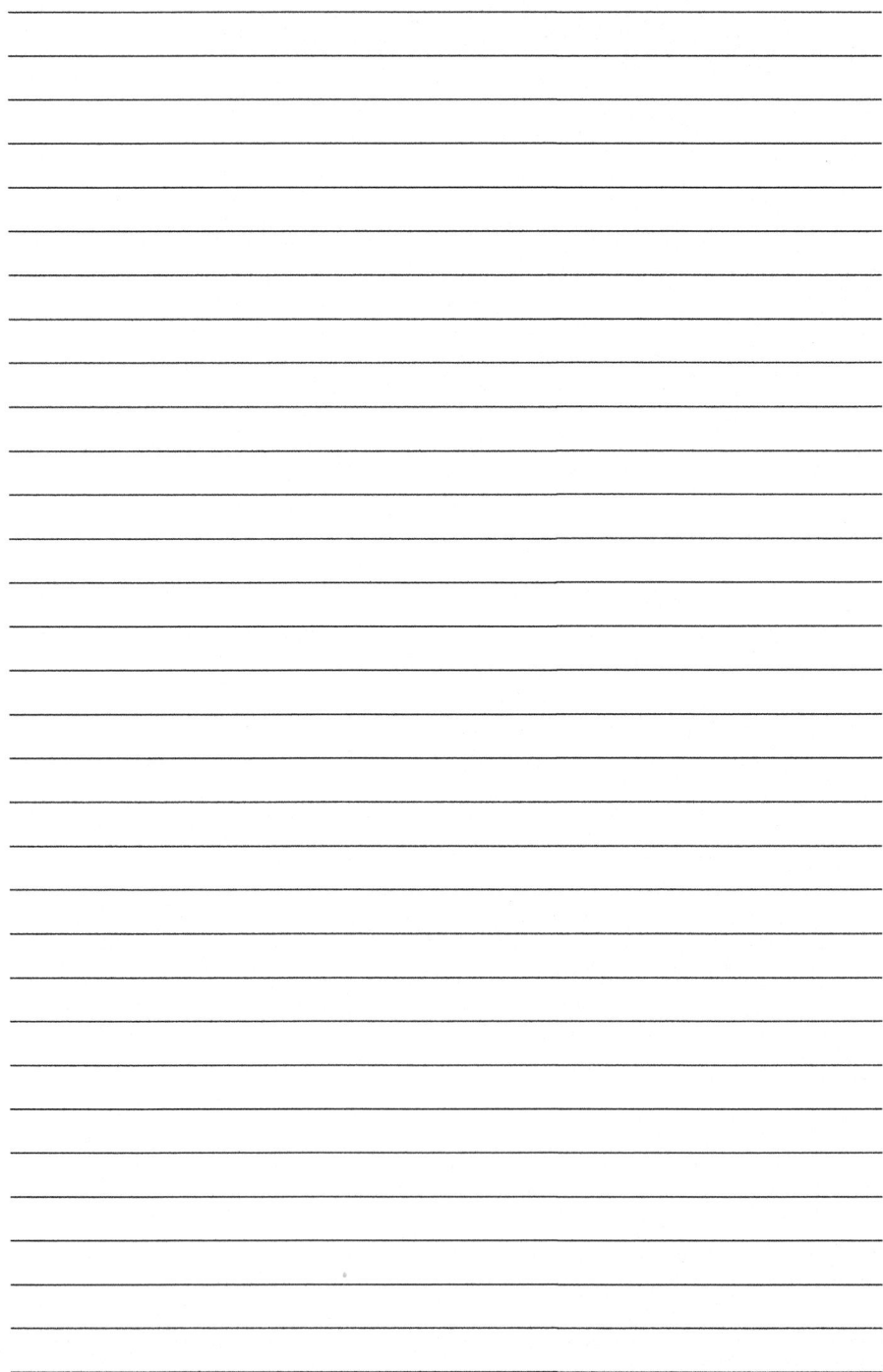

Day 23 Chapter 23
The Power of Play

"We don't stop playing because we grow old; we grow old because we stop playing." - *George Bernard Shaw*

In today's world, dominated by deadlines and demands, the concept of play might seem frivolous or even indulgent. Yet, the significance of play extends far beyond mere entertainment. It's a vital component of human development, creativity, and well-being, transcending age and culture. The ancient Greeks, including Plato, advocated for the integral role of play in education and personal growth, emphasizing its importance not just for children but for society at large. Modern science echoes these ancient philosophies, demonstrating through numerous studies the profound benefits of play for adults as well as children.

Play is not merely a pause from seriousness but a sanctuary of learning and growth. It fosters relaxation and rejuvenation, sparks innovation, and forges connections. Engaging in play can dramatically reduce stress, boost creativity, enhance problem-solving abilities, and improve our interactions with others. The National Institute for Play has highlighted the transformative power of play in enhancing brain function and fueling emotional health, making it a cornerstone for a balanced life.

From the physical exuberance found in a game of soccer to the imaginative realms explored through storytelling, play manifests in myriad forms. Each form serves to enrich our physical vitality, cognitive flexibility, and social bonds. Physical play, such as sports or dancing, not only strengthens our bodies but also releases endorphins, elevating our mood and resilience. Imaginative play, through activities like drawing, acting, or writing, unlocks our creative potential and allows us to explore new perspectives.

Social play, found in board games or collaborative projects, cultivates empathy and teamwork, reinforcing the social fabric that binds us.

Integrating play into our daily routine is not just beneficial—it's essential. Here are five actionable tips to weave play into the tapestry of your life:

- **Dedicate Time for Play:** Actively schedule regular intervals for play in your calendar. Whether it's a weekly sport, a craft project, or a game night with friends, make it a non-negotiable part of your week.
- **Explore New Hobbies:** Use play as an opportunity to explore new interests or revisit past passions. Trying new activities can reinvigorate your mind and body.
- **Incorporate Play at Work:** Introduce playful elements into your workspace or routine, such as brainstorming sessions with creative games or team-building activities that encourage laughter and collaboration.
- **Use Play as a Problem-Solving Tool:** Approach challenges with a playful mindset. Sometimes, the most innovative solutions come from thinking outside the box and engaging with problems in a non-traditional, playful manner.
- **Play with Others:** Engage in social play to strengthen relationships. Shared joy is doubled joy; playing games, sports, or creative projects with others can deepen bonds and build shared memories.

"Play is our brain's favorite way of learning." —*Diane Ackerman*

This ancient activity, revered by both ancestors and modern scientists, is a testament to our innate need for exploration, joy, and connection. By embracing play, we not only enrich our lives but also tap into a wellspring of creativity, resilience, and joy. As we continue on this journey, let's remember to nourish the light wolf within through the powerful, transformative act of play.

Daily Checklist (tick off)

☐ Meditation
☐ 10,000 Steps & Proof
☐ Wolf Workout
☐ Water Intake
☐ 8-Hour Eating Window
☐ Daily Learning (*Homework*)
☐ Supplements (*Optional*)
☐ 7+ Hours of Sleep
☐ Daily Progress Photo
☐ Alcohol & Sugar-Free

Reflect on a moment during this challenge when you felt you surpassed your limits. How can you use that experience to drive you in this final stretch?

_____

_____

_____

_____

How can you adjust your nutrition plan this week to better fuel your intensified workouts?

_____

_____

_____

How are you feeling about your progress as we enter the final stretch of the challenge?

_____

_____

_____

date ___/___/___

Journal the journey

Journal your thoughts on how you feel today and what steps you'll take to succeed tomorrow.

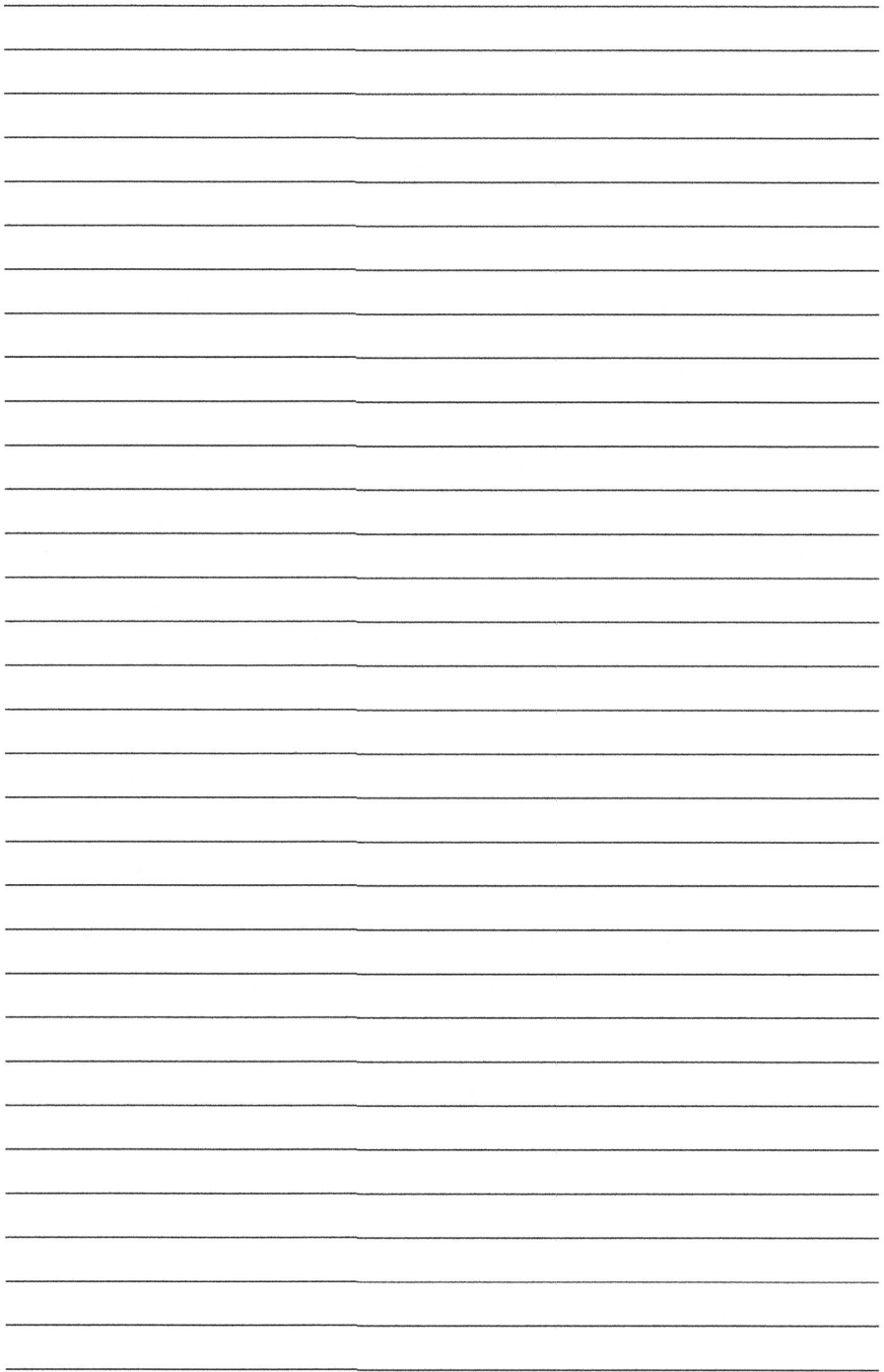

Day 24 Chapter 24
Building endurance & stamina

"Endurance is not just the ability to bear a hard thing, but to turn it into glory." - *William Barclay*

Endurance and stamina are the pillars that support not just physical endeavors but also our resilience in daily life. They are what allow us to thrive under pressure, endure challenges, and emerge stronger. In the timeless words of the ancient philosopher Heraclitus, "Endurance is the first thing that a soldier must possess." This principle holds true beyond the battlefield, extending to every facet of our pursuit of health and well-being.

The journey to enhancing endurance and stamina is multifaceted, integrating physical training, nutrition, hydration, and mental fortitude. It's a testament to the human body's remarkable ability to adapt, grow, and overcome.

Training the Body and Mind

Aerobic Exercise: The foundation of building endurance, aerobic activities like jogging, swimming, and cycling elevate the heart rate, improving the efficiency of the cardiovascular system and thereby extending our ability to sustain activity.

Resistance and Strength Training: Strengthening muscles through resistance training enhances stamina by allowing the body to perform tasks with less perceived effort. Incorporating exercises such as squats, push-ups, and lunges lays the groundwork for muscular endurance.

High-Intensity Interval Training (HIIT): This dynamic approach combines intense bursts of activity with brief rest periods, challenging both aerobic and anaerobic systems, and fostering rapid improvements in endurance and stamina.

Nourishing the Journey

Balanced Nutrition: Fueling the body with the right nutrients is crucial. A diet rich in lean proteins aids muscle repair, complex carbohydrates provide sustained energy, and healthy fats support overall health. Mindful eating, recognizing and responding to the body's hunger cues, ensures optimal fueling for endurance endeavors.

Hydration: Adequate water intake is pivotal for peak performance and recovery. It facilitates nutrient transport, regulates body temperature, and prevents fatigue. The ancient practice of balancing hydration, akin to balancing the body's elemental needs, remains as relevant today as ever.

Mental Resilience

Mental Fortitude: Building endurance and stamina is as much a mental challenge as a physical one. Techniques such as visualization, setting micro-goals, and positive self-talk reinforce mental resilience, empowering us to push beyond perceived limitations.

Rest and Recovery: Acknowledging the role of rest, in harmony with exertion, allows the body and mind to recover and strengthen. This balance is a timeless principle, echoed in the rhythms of nature and human existence.

Embrace Variation: Incorporating a variety of workouts prevents physical and mental burnout, ensuring continuous progress and keeping the journey to improved endurance and stamina both challenging and enjoyable.

"Energy and persistence conquer all things," Benjamin Franklin once remarked, encapsulating the essence of building endurance and stamina. It's a process of continuous effort, guided by wisdom both ancient and modern, and fueled by a relentless pursuit of growth.

In embracing this journey, we unlock our potential, not just as athletes or fitness enthusiasts, but as beings capable of extraordinary perseverance and strength. Let every step taken in endurance be a step towards a fuller, richer experience of life.

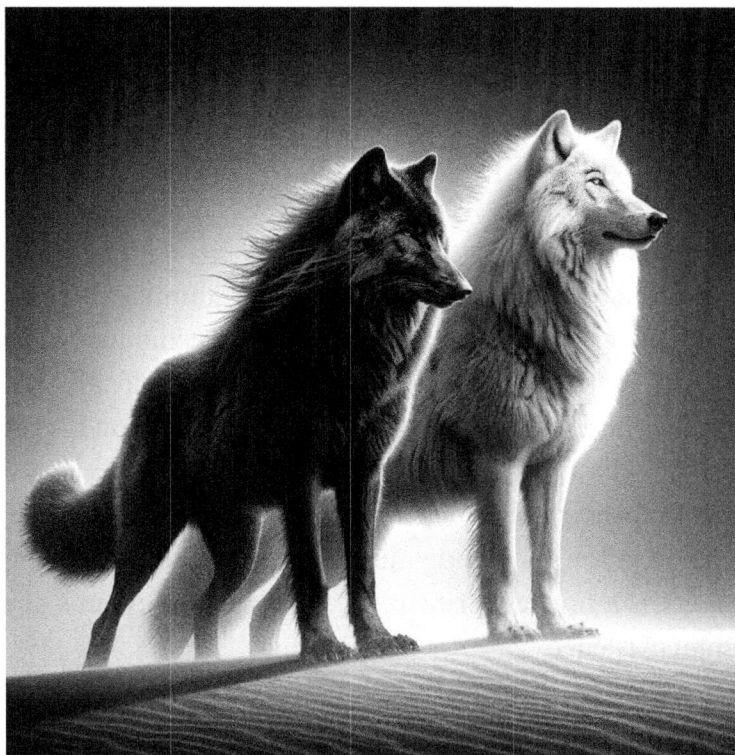

Daily Checklist (tick off)

☐ Meditation
☐ 10,000 Steps & Proof
☐ Wolf Workout
☐ Water Intake
☐ 8-Hour Eating Window
☐ Daily Learning (*Homework*)
☐ Supplements (*Optional*)
☐ 7+ Hours of Sleep
☐ Daily Progress Photo
☐ Alcohol & Sugar-Free

Reflecting on your progress, what specific endurance or stamina goal will you set for the next week?

_____

_____

_____

_____

_____

What's one new habit you've developed during this challenge that you're most proud of?

_____

_____

_____

_____

How has your perspective on physical fitness changed since starting the Two Wolves program?

_____

_____

_____

_____

Journal the journey

Journal your thoughts on how you feel today and what steps you'll take to succeed tomorrow.

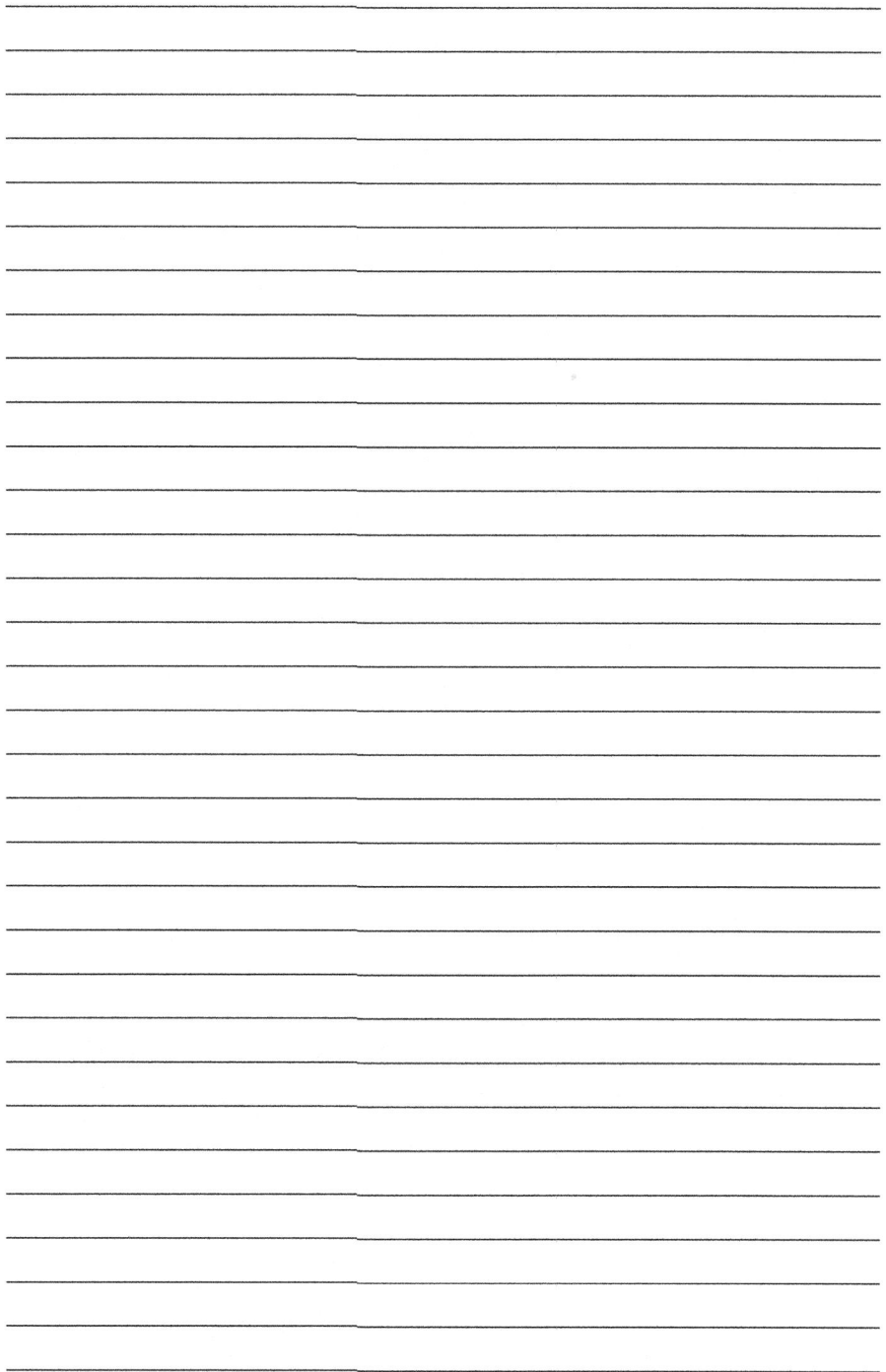

Day 25 Chapter 25
Refining Form & Technique

"Practice doesn't make perfect. Perfect practice makes perfect."
- Vince Lombardi

Refining your form and technique is not merely a matter of physical alignment but a profound journey towards unlocking the full potential of every movement in your fitness journey. Ancient wisdom, echoed by modern scientific findings, underlines the transformative power of attention to detail in every physical endeavor.

Proper form and technique are fundamental not just for efficacy but for safety. Research highlights that correct technique is pivotal in minimizing the risk of injuries, which can range from minor to severe, disrupting one's progress and journey towards fitness (Journal of Strength and Conditioning Research, 2019). Emphasizing form ensures that each movement is executed with precision, engaging the intended muscle groups efficiently while safeguarding joints and ligaments.

Moreover, honing your form and technique significantly enhances performance. The meticulous execution of exercises, such as the squat or deadlift, maximizes muscle engagement and strength development (Clinical Biomechanics, 2018). This focus on form translates into more effective workouts, enabling you to achieve greater results in both strength and endurance.

Enhancing your technique also cultivates confidence. Mastery of form in various exercises not only boosts self-assurance in your fitness capabilities but also enriches your workout experience, fostering a more profound connection with your body and the discipline of physical fitness itself.

To refine your form and technique, consider the following actionable tips:

- **Seek Professional Guidance:** Work with a certified personal trainer or coach who can provide personalized feedback and adjustments to your form.
- **Utilize Visual Aids:** Make use of mirrors in your workout space to self-monitor your form or record your sessions to review and improve.
- **Prioritize Quality Over Quantity:** Focus on performing each repetition with optimal form rather than rushing through sets with improper technique.
- **Engage in Deliberate Practice:** Dedicate sessions specifically to practicing and improving the form of complex exercises, breaking them down into components if necessary.
- **Stay Informed:** Continuously educate yourself on the biomechanics of exercises by consulting reputable sources, including scientific publications and expert-led workshops.

Remember, as the ancient Greeks emphasized through their philosophy and the Olympic spirit, excellence (arete) in any field is achieved through discipline, practice, and continuous refinement. In the words of Aristotle, "*We are what we repeatedly do. Excellence, then, is not an act, but a habit.*" in a modern context as Bruce Lee famously said, "I fear not the man who has practiced 10,000 kicks once, but I fear the man who has practiced one kick 10,000 times." Embrace this philosophy in refining your form and technique; it's the dedication to mastering the fundamentals that build true prowess.

Daily Checklist (tick off)
☐ Meditation
☐ 10,000 Steps & Proof
☐ Wolf Workout
☐ Water Intake
☐ 8-Hour Eating Window
☐ Daily Learning (*Homework*)
☐ Supplements (*Optional*)
☐ 7+ Hours of Sleep
☐ Daily Progress Photo
☐ Alcohol & Sugar-Free

How will you integrate focused practice on form and technique into your next workout session?

_____

_____

_____

_____

_____

What specific exercise do you believe requires your immediate attention to improve its form, and why?

_____

_____

_____

_____

_____

How do you feel as you enter the final week of the challenge, and what steps will you take to ensure you finish strong and apply what you've learned?

_____

_____

_____

_____

date ___ / ___ / ___

Journal the journey

Journal your thoughts on how you feel today and what steps you'll take to succeed tomorrow.

_____
_____
_____
_____
_____
_____
_____
_____
_____
_____
_____
_____
_____
_____
_____
_____
_____
_____
_____
_____
_____
_____
_____
_____
_____
_____
_____
_____
_____
_____
_____
_____

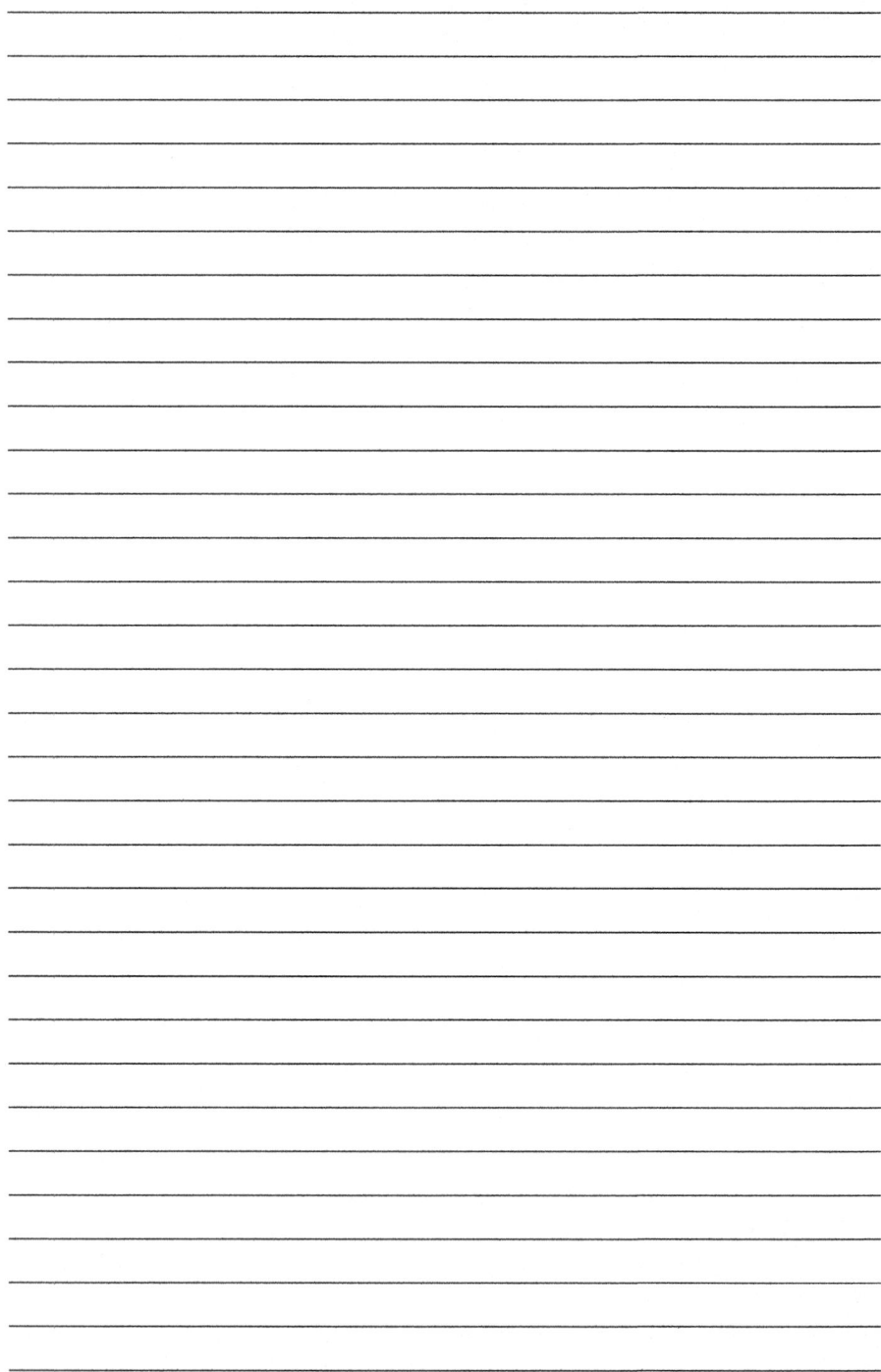

Day 26 Chapter 26
The role of Rest & Recovery

"The innocent sleep, Sleep that knits up the ravell'd sleave of care, The death of each day's life, sore labour's bath, Balm of hurt minds, great nature's second course, Chief nourisher in life's feast."
- *William Shakespeare, Macbeth.*

In a world that often celebrates non-stop productivity and constant activity, the essential nature of rest and recovery remains undervalued. This societal drive towards endless achievement can obscure the fundamental truth that rest and recovery are not just complements to our active endeavors but are foundational to our holistic health and wellness.

Rest and recovery serve as critical periods where our bodies and minds undergo healing, rejuvenation, and strengthening. Physically, when we exert ourselves through exercise or other activities, we create micro-tears in our muscle fibers. It is during the downtime, through processes of rest and recovery, that our bodies repair these micro-tears, leading to stronger and more resilient muscles.

Moreover, rest is paramount for our mental health and cognitive functions. Adequate rest, including quality sleep, plays a significant role in memory consolidation, emotional regulation, and stress management. The importance of mental recovery cannot be overstated, as chronic stress without relief can lead to severe health implications, including, but not limited to, cardiovascular diseases, mental health disorders like anxiety and depression, and impaired immune function.

Quality sleep stands at the forefront of effective rest and recovery strategies. The benefits of sleep extend far beyond mere physical restoration, encompassing critical aspects of mental health, emotional well-being, and cognitive processing. The detriments of sleep deprivation, conversely, can sabotage health, diminish cognitive abilities, and exacerbate stress levels.

In addition to sleep, there are various practices to enhance rest and recovery, including but not limited to, mindful meditation, yoga, and even gentle walking in nature. These activities not only alleviate physical tension but also promote mental clarity and emotional peace.

In embracing rest and recovery, we acknowledge their irreplaceable role in achieving sustained health, vitality, and wellness. As we integrate intentional rest and mindful recovery into our lives, we pave the way for enhanced physical endurance, mental clarity, and a profound sense of well-being.

Actionable Tips:
- **Prioritize Sleep:** Aim for 7-9 hours of quality sleep per night to allow your body and mind to fully recover.
- **Incorporate Relaxation Practices:** Regularly engage in relaxation techniques such as meditation, deep breathing exercises, or yoga to reduce stress and promote mental recovery.
- **Schedule Rest Days:** Include rest days in your fitness regimen to allow your body to repair and strengthen.
- **Stay Hydrated and Nourished:** Ensure you're adequately hydrated and consume a balanced diet to support the recovery process.

- **Listen to Your Body:** Heed your body's signals for rest, and don't push through excessive fatigue or discomfort.

In the words of Leonardo da Vinci, "*Every now and then go away, have a little relaxation, for when you come back to your work your judgment will be surer.*" Let us honor the wisdom of our bodies and minds by embracing the transformative power of rest and recovery.

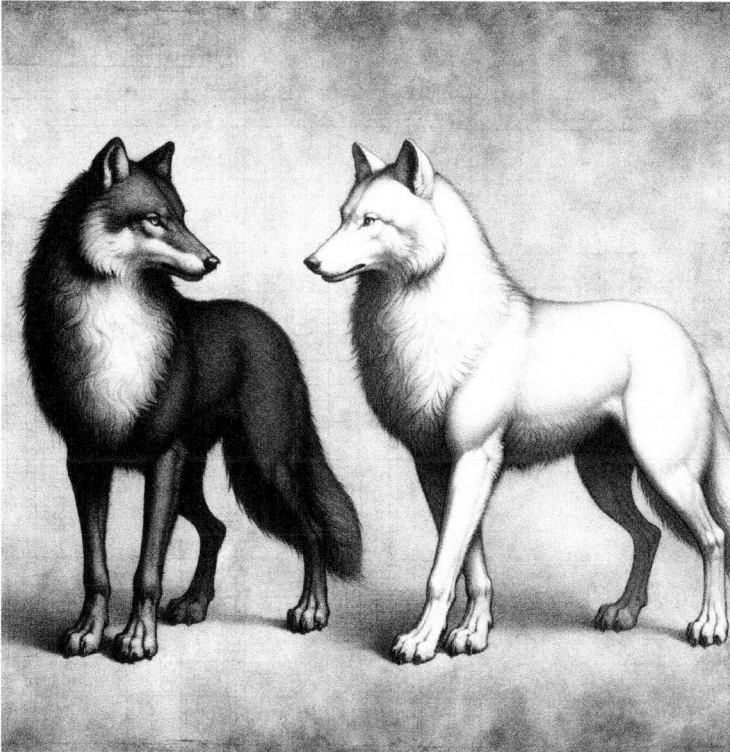

Daily Checklist (tick off)
- ☐ Meditation
- ☐ 10,000 Steps & Proof
- ☐ Wolf Workout
- ☐ Water Intake
- ☐ 8-Hour Eating Window
- ☐ Daily Learning (*Homework*)
- ☐ Supplements (*Optional*)
- ☐ 7+ Hours of Sleep
- ☐ Daily Progress Photo
- ☐ Alcohol & Sugar-Free

What change will you make to your sleep routine to ensure better rest and recovery?

_____

_____

_____

_____

Which relaxation practice (e.g., meditation, yoga) are you committed to incorporating into your daily or weekly schedule?

_____

_____

_____

_____

How has your sleep improved over the course of this challenge, and what changes have you noticed in your daily energy and focus?

_____

_____

_____

_____

date ___ / ___ / ___

Journal the journey

Journal your thoughts on how you feel today and what steps you'll take to succeed tomorrow.

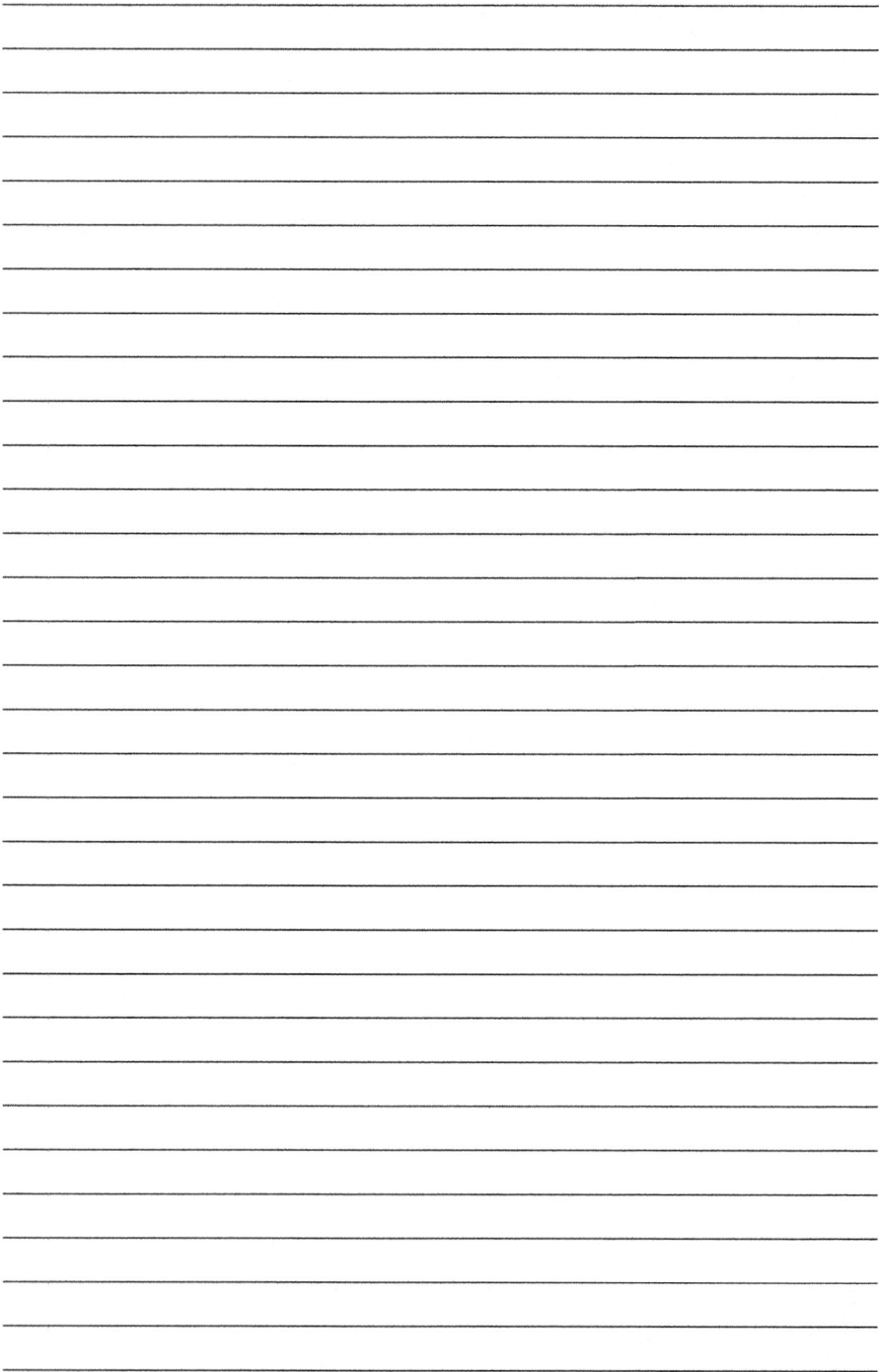

Day 27 Chapter 27
Building on the best version of you

"The privilege of a lifetime is to become who you truly are."
— Carl Jung

As the sun rises, heralding the start of a new day, so too does it signify the dawn of the new you. Over the past few weeks, you've embarked on a transformative journey, guided by the spirit of the Two Wolves and the higher version of yourself. This journey, intricate and profound, has been about much more than physical health or fitness; it's been about reshaping your self-image, about fostering a deep, unwavering belief in your potential and capabilities.

The Journey of Self-Image Transformation
Your self-image is the blueprint of your existence, the core belief system that dictates your actions, your reactions, and the lens through which you view the world and yourself within it. Through the guidance of your spirit wolves, you've challenged this self-image, asking it to evolve, to expand, and to embrace a more positive, empowered version of yourself.

You've faced challenges that once seemed insurmountable, pushed through moments of doubt, and emerged stronger, not just physically, but mentally and spiritually. Each step taken, each barrier overcome, has been a testament to your resilience, your dedication, and your unwavering commitment to growth.

The Higher Version Leading the Way
Your journey has been lit by the beacon of your higher version, the ideal self that embodies all you aspire to be.

This luminous guide has shown you what's possible when you align your actions with your values, when you feed the wolf of positivity, courage, and love, and starve the wolf of fear, doubt, and negativity.

Now, as you stand on this pivotal threshold, you find that your self-image has transformed. You see yourself not as you were, but as you are: stronger, more confident, more capable. This new self-image is a powerful force, propelling you forward, inspiring you to continue your journey towards becoming your best version.

The Ongoing Journey
Yet, it's crucial to remember that the journey doesn't end here. The path to becoming your best version is ongoing, a perpetual cycle of growth, challenge, and transformation. Life will continue to test you, but you now possess the tools, the knowledge, and the spirit to face these tests with grace and strength.

Actionable Tips to Keep Building Your Best Version:
- **Reflect and Reassess:** Regularly take time to reflect on your journey, celebrating your victories and learning from your challenges. Reassess your goals and aspirations to ensure they align with the person you are becoming.
- **Feed Your Spirit Wolves:** Continue to nurture the qualities of your spirit wolves — courage, love, resilience, and wisdom. Let them guide your actions and decisions.
- **Cultivate Positive Relationships:** Surround yourself with people who reflect the version of yourself you wish to become. Their energy, support, and inspiration are invaluable.

- **Embrace Lifelong Learning:** The journey to your best self is one of continuous learning. Seek out new knowledge, experiences, and challenges to foster your growth.
- **Practice Gratitude and Self-Compassion:** Be kind to yourself, recognizing how far you've come. Practice gratitude for your experiences, for they have shaped you into who you are.

The journey is never over, but each step is a step closer to your best version. The version that was always within you, waiting to be discovered, nurtured, and celebrated. Continue to walk this path with pride, determination, and an open heart. The best is yet to come.

"The only person you are destined to become is the person you decide to be." — Ralph Waldo Emerson

This journey is yours, and yours alone. Embrace it, cherish it, and walk it with the wisdom of the wolves guiding you home.

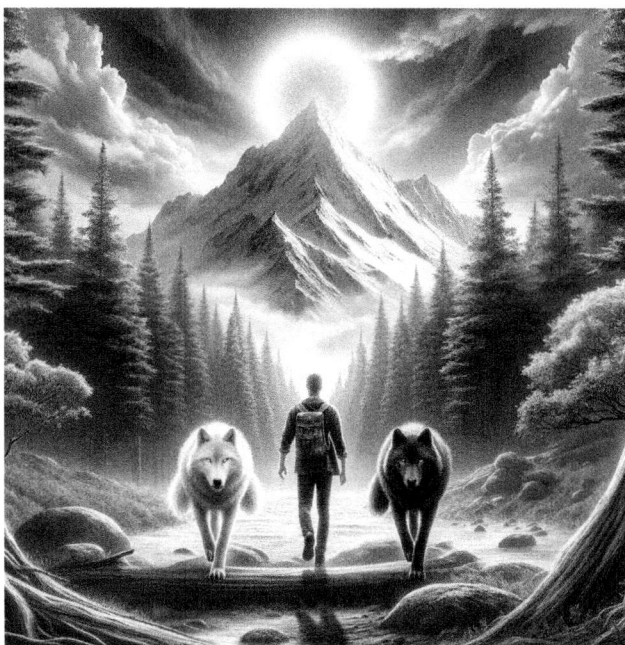

Daily Checklist (tick off)

☐ Meditation
☐ 10,000 Steps & Proof
☐ Wolf Workout
☐ Water Intake
☐ 8-Hour Eating Window
☐ Daily Learning (*Homework*)
☐ Supplements (*Optional*)
☐ 7+ Hours of Sleep
☐ Daily Progress Photo
☐ Alcohol & Sugar-Free

How has your self-image evolved throughout this journey, and in what ways do you see yourself differently now?

_____

_____

_____

_____

_____

What aspects of your higher self have you discovered and nurtured during this program?

_____

_____

_____

_____

As you look ahead, what steps will you take to continue building and living as the best version of yourself?

_____

_____

_____

_____

Journal the journey

Journal your thoughts on how you feel today and what steps you'll take to succeed tomorrow.

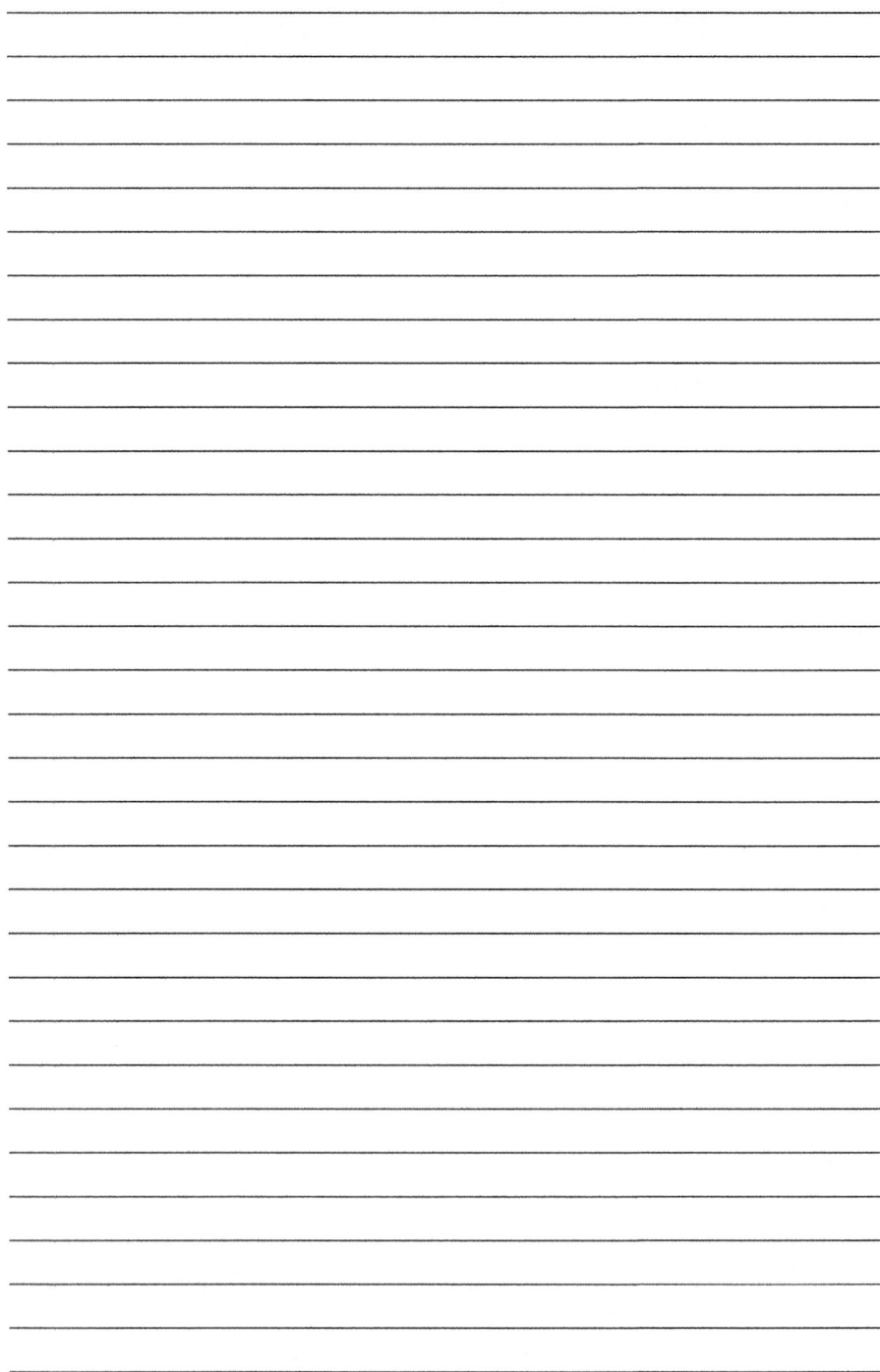

Day 28 Chapter 28
Maintaining Momentum

"Success is a journey, not a destination." - *Oscar Wilde*

You stand on the threshold of a transformative moment, not just marking the end of a 30-day journey, but also the beginning of a new chapter in your life. As you transition from the disciplined structure of this program into the vastness of everyday life, the real challenge begins: maintaining your progress and scaling new heights. This isn't merely about fitness; it's about crafting a lifestyle that resonates with vitality, resilience, and joy. Let's delve into actionable strategies to carry forward the momentum you've built, ensuring that your achievements are not just milestones but stepping stones to greater wellness and fulfillment.

- **Embrace Incremental Progress:** The essence of enduring success lies in celebrating every small victory and learning from each setback. Modern research underscores the power of incremental progress in sustaining motivation and enhancing satisfaction across life's domains (Clear, 2018). Begin each day with a simple question: "*What small step can I take today to improve my well-being?*" This approach keeps the journey towards wellness dynamic and adaptable.
- **Cultivate a Mindful Routine Mindfulness:** the art of being fully present and engaged in the moment, can transform the mundane into the extraordinary. Applying mindfulness to your daily routine, from savoring your meals to being fully immersed in your workouts, enhances both the quality and the enjoyment of these experiences. Studies in behavioral psychology have shown that mindfulness can significantly reduce stress and improve quality of life (Kabat-Zinn, 1994).

- **Harness the Power of Community:** The journey towards lifelong fitness is enriched by the company we keep. Surround yourself with a community that shares your aspirations and values. Whether it's joining a local fitness group, participating in online forums, or simply engaging with friends on similar paths, the support and motivation of a community are invaluable. Social support has been scientifically linked to better health outcomes and sustained behavior change (Uchino, 2006).
- **Stay Curious and Keep Learning:** Your growth shouldn't stop as this program concludes. Stay curious about your health and well-being by exploring new activities, reading up on the latest fitness and nutrition research, and experimenting with different ways to stay active and nourished. Lifelong learning is not just about acquiring knowledge; it's about staying engaged, excited, and energized about your health journey.
- **Set New Horizons:** As you've reached this milestone, it's time to look ahead and set new goals. Reflect on what you've learned about yourself, identify areas you're passionate about improving, and commit to new objectives. Whether it's mastering a complex yoga pose, running a half marathon, or achieving a new level of mental clarity and emotional resilience, let your ambitions evolve as you do.

Remember: You're not at the end; you're at a beginning. The last 30 days have been a foundation, a launchpad into a lifestyle where fitness, wellness, and happiness are interwoven into the fabric of your daily life. As you step into the future, carry with you the lessons learned, the strength gained, and the confidence earned. You've shed the wolf cub's puppy fat to reveal the Omega within - a symbol of your evolved, empowered self, ready to navigate the complexities of life with grace, strength, and an unquenchable thirst for growth. Here's to the journey ahead - may it be as rewarding as the path you've already traversed.

Daily Checklist (tick off)

☐ Meditation
☐ 10,000 Steps & Proof
☐ Wolf Workout
☐ Water Intake
☐ 8-Hour Eating Window
☐ Daily Learning (*Homework*)
☐ Supplements (*Optional*)
☐ 7+ Hours of Sleep
☐ Daily Progress Photo
☐ Alcohol & Sugar-Free

What habit developed during this challenge do you find most valuable for your future?

_____

_____

_____

_____

_____

Reflecting on your journey, what's one lesson you'll carry with you?

_____

_____

_____

_____

_____

How do you feel? Simple question for some, difficult for others...

_____

_____

_____

_____

_____

_____

_____

date ___ / ___ / ___

Journal the journey

Journal your thoughts on how you feel today and what steps you'll take to succeed tomorrow.

Becoming Omega

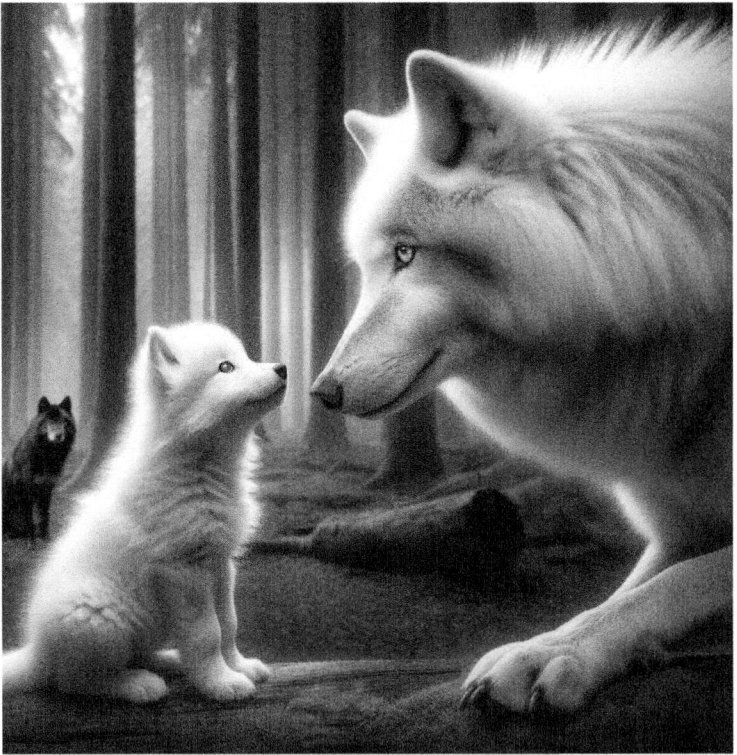

A cub no more...

Day 29 Chapter 29
Only the beginning...

"The journey of a thousand miles begins with one step." - *Lao Tzu*

You stand on the precipice of a remarkable achievement, a day away from completing a transformative 30-day journey with the Two Wolves program. Reflect on the person you were when you began this journey and who you have become. This transformation, this renewed sense of vitality and strength, is a testament to your dedication, resilience, and the power of positive change.

However, let's not view this as the end but rather a pivotal beginning. The habits you've nurtured and the lessons learned are stepping stones to a lifelong pursuit of wellness and personal growth. To support you in continuing this journey, we're thrilled to introduce you to the Omega phase—a 60-day challenge designed to elevate your achievements and solidify your transformation.

Elevating Your Journey: The Omega Phase
The Omega phase isn't just an extension of this program; it's an elevation. Here, you'll engage with more advanced strategies, continue to grow within our supportive community, and embrace challenges that refine your resilience and determination.

Actionable Tips for Transitioning into Omega and what to expect:
- **Set New, Challenging Goals:** Reflect on your achievements and outline new goals that push your limits. Whether it's improving your personal best, mastering a new fitness skill, or enhancing mental resilience, let your aspirations guide you.
- **Deepen Your Knowledge:** Use the next two days to dive deeper into areas you wish to explore further. Whether it's nutrition, mindfulness, or advanced training techniques, knowledge is power.

- **Prepare Mentally and Physically:** The Omega phase demands more from you. Begin integrating more intense sessions and mindfulness practices into your routine to prepare both your body and mind.
- **Connect with the Community:** Share your journey, your upcoming transition, and seek out Omega veterans for advice and inspiration. Remember, you are part of a pack, and together, we thrive.
- **Embrace the Omega Mindset:** Start every day with the mantra, "I am Omega." Let this be a reminder of your strength, your journey, and the endless possibilities that lie ahead.

Remember, what you've started here is a lifelong journey of growth and self-improvement. As you prepare for the final stretch, push yourself harder than ever before—let the Omega within you roar with determination and strength. Awooo!

In the words of Confucius, "*It does not matter how slowly you go as long as you do not stop.*" As you step into the Omega phase, carry forward this spirit of perseverance and unyielding progress.

Ready to embrace the challenge and reveal your Omega self? A new horizon awaits, filled with opportunities to push your limits and redefine your potential. Let's continue this journey together. Awooo!

Engage, Elevate, Embrace: Your Omega Journey Begins Now.

Daily Checklist (tick off)

☐ Meditation
☐ 10,000 Steps & Proof
☐ Wolf Workout
☐ Water Intake
☐ 8-Hour Eating Window
☐ Daily Learning (*Homework*)
☐ Supplements (*Optional*)
☐ 7+ Hours of Sleep
☐ Daily Progress Photo
☐ Alcohol & Sugar-Free

Reflecting on the journey so far, what has been your most significant realization about yourself?

_____
_____
_____
_____
_____

How has your perspective on personal growth and fitness transformed throughout this program?

_____
_____
_____
_____
_____

Are you ready for the Omega phase? How much rest will you need before taking yourself to the next phase?

_____
_____
_____
_____
_____
_____
_____

Journal the journey

Journal your thoughts on how you feel today and what steps you'll take to succeed tomorrow.

_____
_____
_____
_____
_____
_____
_____
_____
_____
_____
_____
_____
_____
_____
_____
_____
_____
_____
_____
_____
_____
_____
_____
_____
_____
_____
_____
_____
_____
_____
_____
_____
_____
_____

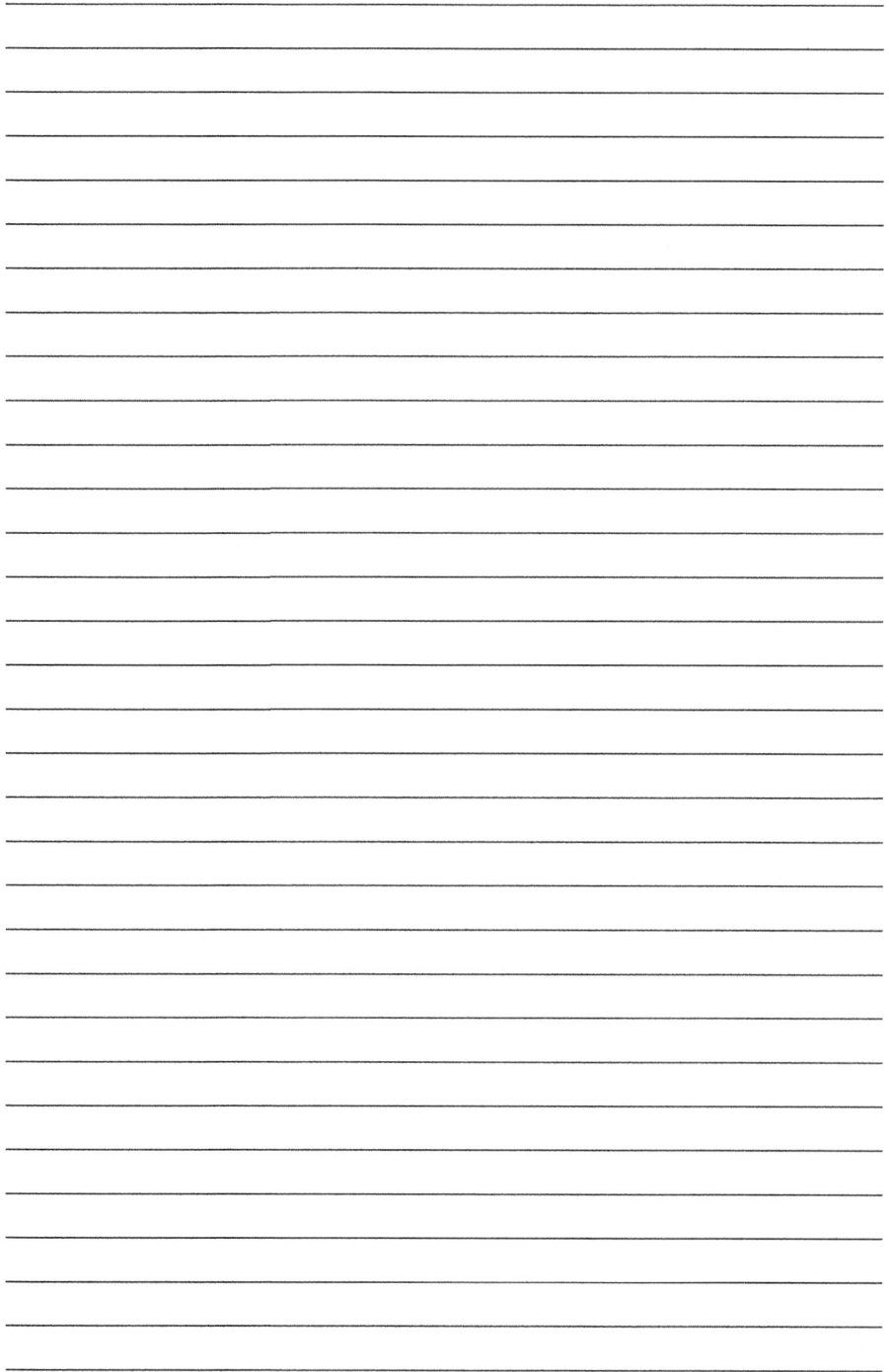

Day 30 Chapter 30
Omega Unleashed: Beyond the Horizon

"Every new beginning comes from some other beginning's end."
– Seneca

You have completed the 30-day Two Wolves program, and you are no longer a wolf cub. You have gained valuable knowledge, skills, and experience in taking back control of your life and creating a positive mindset.

You have come a long way, and you should be proud of yourself! In just 30 days, you have learned how to resist the dark wolf, build resilience, manage stress, strengthen your support network, advance your fitness level, refine your technique, and maintain your progress.

You have overcome challenges and obstacles, and you have grown stronger and wiser. But this is only the beginning of your journey. The Omega phase of the Two Wolves program is waiting for you. This is a 60-day challenge that will take you even further on your positive journey.

In the Omega phase, you will face new challenges, learn new skills, and connect with a community of like-minded people who share your goals and values. The Omega phase will challenge you to push beyond your limits and discover your full potential.

The Two Wolves program is not just a 30-day or 60-day challenge. It is a way of life. It is a philosophy of growth, transformation, and empowerment. It is a journey of self-discovery, self-improvement, and self-actualization.

It is a path that leads to a better, stronger, and happier you. So, dear reader, I encourage you to take the next step and join the Omega phase of the Two Wolves program.

Find the links at the back of the book to find out more and sign up. This is your chance to continue your positive journey and become the best version of yourself. Remember, you have the power to choose which wolf to feed.

Choose wisely and keep moving forward! Congratulations once again on completing the 30-day Two Wolves program.

You are not a wolf cub anymore, but a wise and strong wolf.

"Keep howling and see you in the next phase of your journey!"
Hunter W.J.

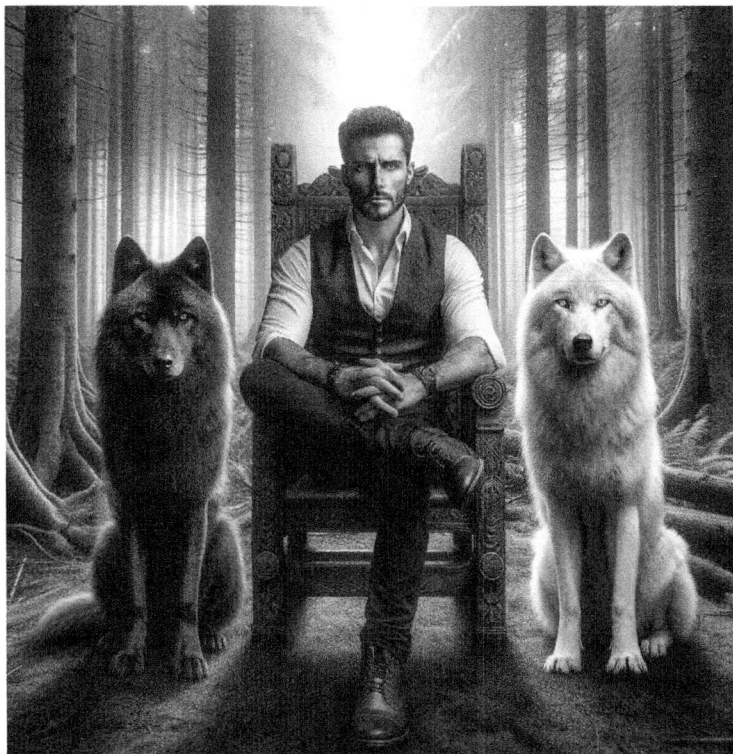

date ___ / ___ / ___

Journal the journey

Journal your thoughts on how you feel today and what steps you'll take to succeed tomorrow.

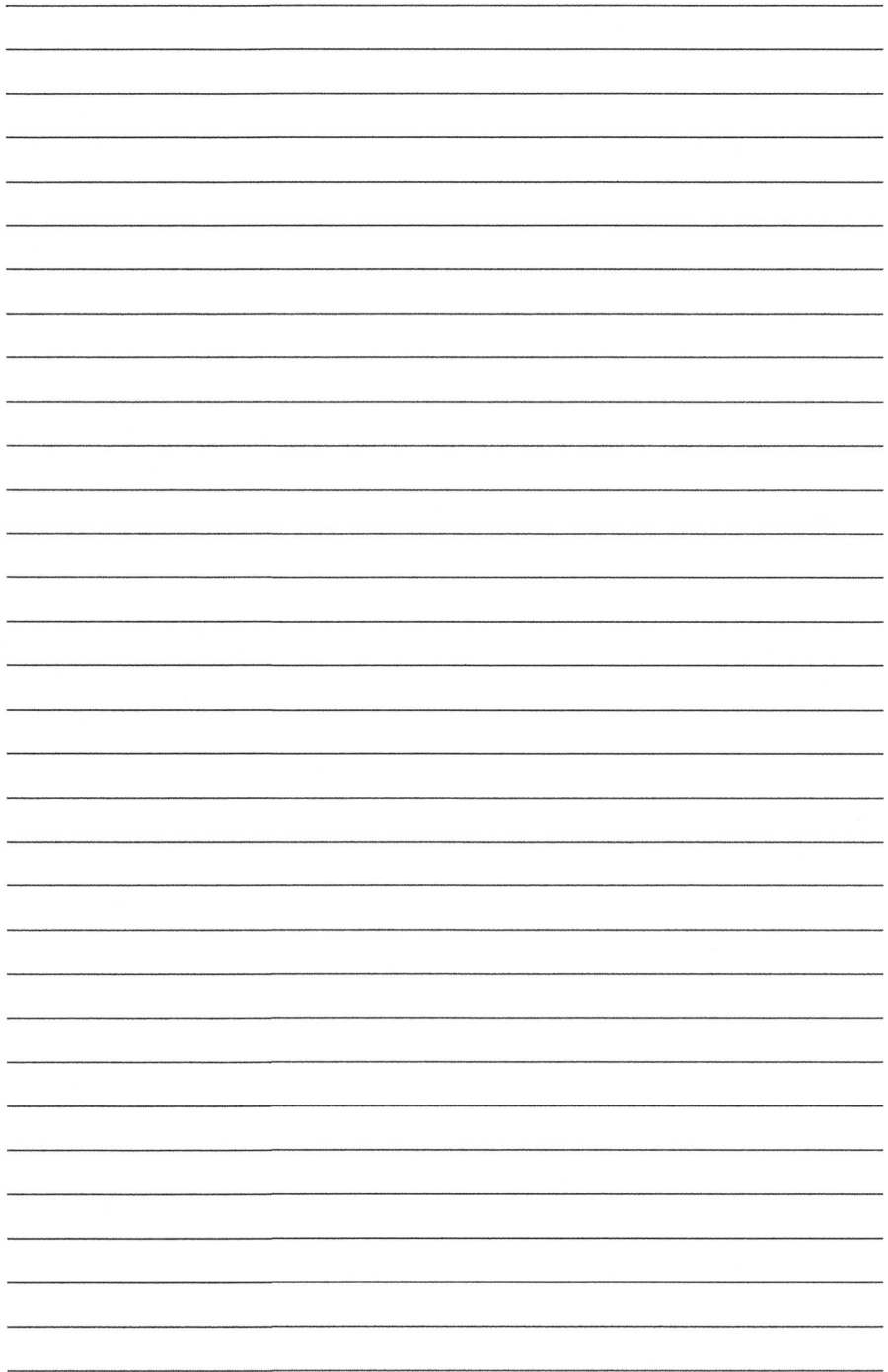

Biomarker Measurements

Date of Measurement: _____

_____ | **Weight**: Morning measurement before eating (lbs/kg).

_____ | **Body Fat %:** Use a scale or caliper (%).

_____ | **Waist Circumference**: Measure above the belly button (inches/cm).

_____ | **Bicep Circumference:** Measure the fullest part of the bicep (inches/cm).

_____ | **Thigh Circumference:** Measure the fullest part of the thigh (inches/cm).

_____ | **Resting Heart Rate:** Measure upon waking, count beats for 60 seconds (bpm).

_____ | **Blood Pressure:** Use a blood pressure monitor (mmHg).

_____ | **Touch Toes:** Can you touch your toes? Note the distance if not (Yes/No/Distance).

_____ | **Mood:** Rate on a scale of 1 being very poor mood, 10 being excellent (1-10 scale).

Instructions: Fill in the blanks with your initial measurements to establish a baseline for your progress. This structured approach allows you to monitor improvements and adapt your journey as needed, fostering a path toward holistic wellness.

Links to join the pack

Find everything here
https://linktr.ee/twowolvescollective

Facebook
facebook.com/2wolvescollective
Instagram
@two.wolves.collective
YouTube
youtube.com/@TwoWolvesCollective

Continue your journey...

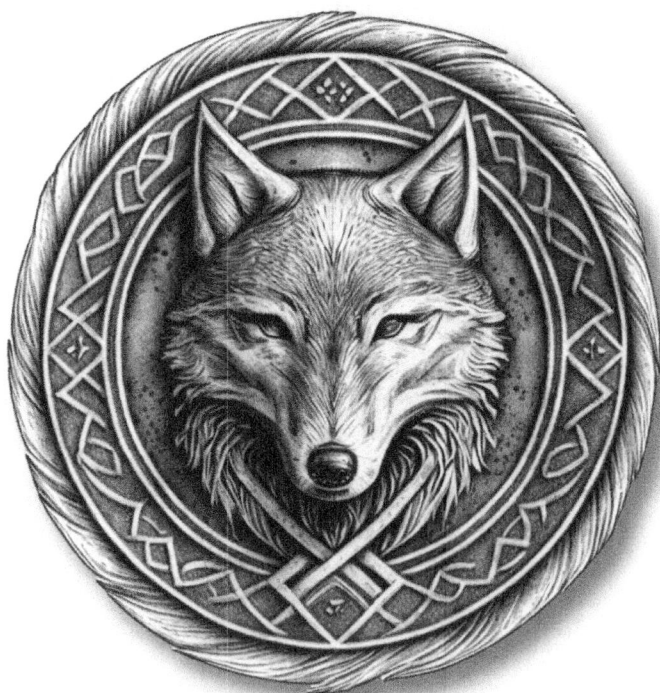

Join the Omega pack

Printed in Great Britain
by Amazon

40980735R00169